Tantric Awakening

Tantric Awakening

A Woman's Initiation
into the Path of Ecstasy

Valerie Brooks

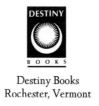

Destiny Books
Rochester, Vermont

Destiny Books
One Park Street
Rochester, Vermont 05767
www.InnerTraditions.com

Destiny Books is a division of Inner Traditions International

Library of Congress Cataloging-in-Publication Data

Brooks, Valerie.
    Tantric awakening : a woman's initiation into the path of ecstasy / Valerie Brooks.
        p. cm.
    ISBN 0-89281-906-5 (pbk.)
    1. Sex instruction. 2. Tantrism. 3. Sex—Religious aspects—Tantrism. I. Title.
    HQ64 .B76 2001

2001005264

Printed and bound in Canada

10 9 8 7 6 5 4 3 2

Text design and layout by Rachel Goldenberg
This book was typeset in Deepdene and Charme as the display typeface

To Jim,

my mentor, inspiration,

and best friend.

This book is also dedicated to my fellow Americans. The terrorism of September 11, 2001 is what anger and hatred within the human heart are capable of. But in this aftermath we also witness the triumph of good: we are heroes, survivors, and a nation more united than ever. It is my hope that this day forever reminds us to look within ourselves and transcend our rage, self-destruction, and hatred. May justice and peace prevail on Earth.

Contents

Part 3

Tantra and Community

Part 4

Path of God

Acknowledgements

Many thanks to the staff of Inner Traditions for their assistance and effort, especially Jon Graham, for believing in me; Jeanie Levitan, for your wisdom and collaborative style; Doris Troy for your great ability to fine tune; and Lee Awbrey, for your perceptive understanding of me and this book, and for gently guiding me through all the details.

I would also like to thank all of my friends who have supported me through the writing of *Tantric Awakening*. A true friend is someone who is willing to be there when times are really rough and when times are great beyond imagination. To all of my true friends, I am eternally grateful for your presence in my life and your unending support.

Namaste.

Introduction

*T*antra, the art of spiritual sexuality, has been teasing us lately. Late-night news segments and sexy magazine covers report that it can spice up our sex life better than Viagra, improve our health more than herbs, and awaken the flame of personal enlightenment. But few explain why, or how. Even those providing good academic instructions fail to mention what really ends up happening to the serious student of tantra. Can its benefits be realized by anyone? Or is tantra merely an excuse for sexual indulgence?

I can tell you from eleven years of personal experience that the promises of tantra are real, for I am living them. And indeed, as teasingly suggested, this sweet yoga of love is *really* fun. When I discovered tantra at the ripe young age of nineteen, I had no idea how it was to affect my physical body, transform my emotions, or even create the occasional perils that I had to face. By using my sexuality to facilitate higher states of consciousness, I found answers to fundamental questions: What do I really want? Where is my true happiness found? Where am *I* found?

Sexual essence is the most powerful energy available to us on a personal level. This force that ignites the miracle of life can also be used to elevate physical, emotional, and spiritual consciousness. Tantra is not a religion; it is ber that sweet flame of desire within you: the fire that beckons you to know your essence and source of unending happiness. Come with me now, and look inside my life: a tantrika's life, ignited through tantra. Let me tell you what really happens if you should ever be so bold as to dip your toes, or plunge your entire being, into this path of ecstasy.

Part 1
Physical Elation

Falling in Love 1

lames rise from my pelvis, licking my heart, playing my body with deep hues of red that melt into orange and yellow, then cool me with green, blue, violet. An orgasm of color, the boundaries of my skin blur fuzzy, and the pleasure dances now outside of my body, taking me with it, so that I become the ecstasy that lives in the ether surrounding me.

Stubborn, that's what I am. Stubbornness kept me from siding with either faction of my divorced family. Stubbornness kept me from blindly accepting the values of my generation. And now, as I lie here, barely able to breathe, I thank God for my stubbornness.

My senses are dancing. Currents of hot and cool energy swim up and down my spine, pouring into my loins and out the tips of my fingers. These few hours have passed like moments. Content in my partner's arms, I read his body, feel his feelings, and know his thoughts. Our bodies feel merged into one luxuriant energy of bliss.

I feel like a goddess—transcendent and linked with every woman, past, present, and future. I am the seductress, lover, mother, sister, and caretaker. My heart sings with a compassion for all people and things that make up this miraculous world.

Opening my eyes, I turn to my partner, and a laugh escapes my buzzing lips. *Wow! How did we do that?* With a smile he teases, "This is only the beginning."

For several hours I have been absorbed in meditation. I have not been sitting silently alone in lotus position; I have been breathing, feeling, and sensing—in oneness—between the sheets of my bed with my partner. The ecstatic feelings I now encounter, which begin through the simple exercises of tantra, have positively affected every aspect of my life.

Tantra taught me how to master my emotions and go beyond my fear, fertilizing the seeds of self-confidence that had been buried for years. My emotional outlook transformed from insecurity and self-doubt to a high self-esteem and certainty. Tantra helped me put my destiny into my own hands.

My creativity blossomed. Every part of my day—from mundane dishwashing, to the routine of work, to my highest artistic aspirations— became an experience of joy, symmetry, and oneness. Every moment became an opportunity to grow and to express myself.

Struggles with money vanished. Prosperity, like a flowing river, poured into my life. I embraced what it means to feel truly supported by the universe. I healed family relationships that had been damaged for years. My friendships and loving relationships became increasingly more fulfilling. Letting go of desperation, negative thinking, and self-hatred, I learned what "unconditional love" really means.

My perception of spirituality and God took on an entirely different meaning, one that was founded on experience rather than hearsay, choice rather than indoctrination. I began to release everything inside me that was not in harmony with my essence. Tantra became my passageway to a destiny built upon total choice, a destiny that would link me to an ever increasing love for self and others.

But who I am today is not who I was eleven years ago when I first discovered tantra. During the fateful summer that marked the beginning of my destiny with tantra, I was, one could say, quite a head case.

Beginnings

My emotions dominated my life. I wore depression like a comfortable bathrobe, and worry, its close cousin, clung my side. "You're so moody," my family would tell me. Had my parents not been adverse to antidepressants, I might have been medicated for the severe mood swings I suffered.

My past is not different from that of many other people of my generation. In the middle-class suburb in California where I grew up, we learned that looking good on the outside was more important than feeling good on the inside. Our happy exteriors hid eating disorders and extreme insecurity. We might have been the poster children for low self-esteem. Yet we had power. We had at our fingertips every possible piece of information (and substance) with which to do whatever we chose. We thought we knew everything. We all wanted to belong to something great: a something we didn't quite understand.

My broken family was also typically dysfunctional. As the youngest of six children, I figured that if I did everything right I could make up for the mistakes of the whole family and rescue everyone from all past mistakes and pain. I tried really hard to get it all "right." I got straight A's in school in an attempt to gain my parents' attention. I wanted them to notice me: the shy girl in the corner who had so much to say but lacked the nerve. I tried cheerleading, gymnastics, softball, and diving—all terrible choices for me, an inherent klutz. (I usually won the "most improved" award for starting out hopelessly bad and not giving up in the face of humiliation!) Theater was a great outlet, as it gave me the approval that I desperately needed (and it required much less physical coordination!). But despite all my experimentation, nothing seemed to satisfy an inner yearning that I could hardly define. One remnant of my parents' divorce was the conflicting message I received about God. My father's side of the family was comprised of born-again Christian extremists. Joint custody dictated that every other weekend, come Sunday, we would all pack into Dad's van and head off to church, singing hymns and reciting prayers. Following the footsteps of my revered stepsisters, I devoutly accepted Christianity at the early age of nine, vowing that I would spend my life serving God. I liked the structure and discipline of a strong spiritual life.

But the messages of Christianity, although fundamentally good, left me with many unanswered questions. Why are we intrinsically sinful, even from birth? Why is my sexuality bad? Why does God send non-Christians to hell? The responses and sermons of the pastors did not always stand up to scrutiny.

My mother's household, which is where I spent the majority of my childhood, embraced the other extreme. Mom's family was spiritual, but not religious. According to them, one's relationship with God is personal. Church was not a consideration, even during religious holidays. Mom was wise in a down-to-earth way.

"Heaven and hell are right here on Earth," she would say. To her, spirituality was simply one part of life. Books on all types of philosophies could be found, especially in my eldest brother's room. There I would learn of Eastern religions, astrology, and metaphysical subjects from authors such as Jack Kerouac, Linda Goodman, and Herman Hesse.

I liked my mother's practical and self-reliant sense of spirituality, but I wanted more. Not knowing it at the time, I was seeking a path that I had yet to fully comprehend.

And so at nineteen I was open to a different way of looking at things. My first year away from home at an eastern college had done nothing for my self-esteem. I had gained the perfunctory "college twenty," my face was a mess of acne, and, as usual, I was sexually frustrated (the all-women's college didn't help). Above all, I didn't know who I really was, and I finally felt courageous (or confused) enough to find out. One early-summer day, I simply said a prayer. I asked God to show me what I was looking for. Less than one month later I discovered tantra.

A New Path

Early that summer I was invited by a friend to a rebirthing workshop* at a local bookstore. Searching for answers to questions I couldn't even articulate, I jumped at the opportunity, and found myself sitting in a large circle of about thirty people in an incense-filled room on a warm Friday evening. A

*Rebirthing is a spiritual technique discovered by Leonard Orr and Sondra Roy. It is also known as conscious breathing.

couple walked in the door a half hour late, disturbing our silent meditation. The instructor rolled his eyes as we all looked in their direction. For some reason my heart skipped a beat. *A vague memory . . . some kind of connection . . .* It was unexplainable.

Thus interrupted, the instructor asked us to do one exercise before beginning the rebirthing. We were first to choose a partner. I turned to the woman behind me who had just arrived. When I looked into her deep brown eyes, I felt I knew her from lifetimes ago. Later I discovered that she and her husband were tantric teachers. They had been ordained by the Kriya Jyoti Tantra Society of Southern India.*

The instructor asked us to share an issue we were coping with and our goals for its resolution. Our partners were to support us by replying, "I support you and I want that for you." I told my partner that I wanted to lose the twenty pounds I had gained the previous year. When she looked into my eyes and said, quietly but firmly, "I want that for you," it was as though I had remembered her saying that many, many times before.

I didn't know anything about tantra then. I didn't even know that the woman and her husband were tantric teachers. But over the two weeks following the workshop the extra weight dropped from me as though by miracle, and their faces lingered in my mind.

Blessing in Disguise

For reasons beyond my control, I was unable to go back to college in the fall. My father had lost his job, and I couldn't get funding to pay for the following year. My attraction to tantra was so strong that I decided to take off one year to study this subject in great detail.

Over the course of that year I studied many spiritual books, such as *A Course in Miracles.*[†] Despite my impatient nature, from age nineteen to twenty-one I didn't actually practice any tantra.[‡] Taking the advice of my new teachers, I decided first to understand it and then to prepare my mind

---

*The Varma Mara path of tantra kriya yoga, Saraswati order.

[†] *A Course in Miracles* (Tiburon, Calif.: Foundation for Inner Peace, 1996).

[‡] Hereinafter, *tantra* refers to the act of tantric lovemaking, or tantric sex.

and body by doing other disciplines. I practiced rebirthing, meditation, prayer, Kriya yoga,* and fasting.

After one year, I was still unable to come up with funding for my private college, so I decided to transfer to a school in California. I studied with my teachers in the form of counseling sessions (their primary business, unrelated to tantra, was helping people through personal and relationship counseling). These sessions helped me work through some very large emotional issues. And tantra, well, what can I say? Tantra seduced me with its silent beckoning. Although I did not attempt to begin this mysterious calling, it continued to intrigue me. My teachers taught me more about tantra from their actions than from their words. Their honesty, depth of character, immense love for others, and giving nature were a lesson unto itself for me. Never had I met such a spiritually gifted man and woman before. A sweet peace emanated from their presence, and everyone around them felt it. Tantra, I learned, utilizes a tremendous amount of energy, and its beneficial effects will shine when the practitioner is fully ready to accept this energy. It is a bit like stretching before a vigorous workout.

This time of intensive study and personal reflection also allowed me to get over the initial lusting fascination that I had with tantra. Part of me wanted to use tantra to rebel. It would have been a bandage to cover up my disillusionment with religion and would also be something that my family would never understand—sort of a rebellious affront to their beliefs. But one needs a clear head and clear agenda for starting a path of tantra, and it took me some time to get there.

Yet, having chosen tantra (or perhaps it chose me), everything in my life began to fall into place. I had become a student—not just of academics, but also of spirituality. I had begun the first steps in exploring every aspect of myself through this ancient art of tantra.

*Kriya yoga emphasizes the breath and visualization of energy.

Tantra

Tantra, beloved word, is first discovered in Sanskrit.* It comes from *tanoti,* "to expand," and *trayati,* "liberation." *Tantra* also means "to weave," as if to weave together the community, or to weave the hearts of people into one. Tantra, considered the yoga of love, is also called tantra yoga.†

Tantra's roots are in Hindu and Buddhist sects of India, where today it is practiced in limited areas just as it was traditionally practiced a thousand years ago. Known by many different names, tantra has been affected by, and has directly influenced, some religious groups of China and Japan. In China tantra's precepts are seen in Taoism, where sex is used to achieve spiritual happiness as well as physical energy and longevity. In Japan, some sects of Buddhism practice tantra. Yet tantra can be traced back to early peoples, and its essence is found in almost all societies. Any celebration of the creative life force is tantric in nature.

Tantra is not a religion. It doesn't require adopting a spiritual belief system or adhering to doctrines. Tantra can be a positive complement to any existing lifestyle or religion. Tantra can also be the foundation of one's life. It is flexible enough to complement and strong enough to uphold. Tantra is a way. Its methodology automatically causes the experience of enlightenment, or truth, or God, regardless of one's faith. Tantra can be learned as a specific set of instructions, but its nature is fluid. Like any form of art or creation, tantra's expression is uniquely personal. It cannot be separated from the individual practioner.

In tantra I found a synergy between sexuality and spirituality, between tradition and spontaneity, between the communal and the subjective. It was like glue to me. It brought together all the seemingly irreconcilable pieces, merging the contradictory and disparate messages of religion, philosophy, and literature. Tantra guided me inward, showing me that my darkest demons were illusions built of dust. In essence, it enabled me to become a completely different person.

*Sanskrit is one of the most ancient written languages.

†Other branches of yoga include asthanga (raja)—from which the popular hatha yoga movement originates—bhakti, karma, jnana, kundalini, and kriya.

The human heart is a miracle. It makes heroes of us. It helps us love others more than we love ourselves. It gives us patience and strength to endure the many hardships of our lives. It is the reason that soldiers sacrifice their lives. It is the reason we go beyond our judgmental minds and forgive the crimes against us. Our hearts make us bigger than we are. Our hearts are our everlasting link to whatever we think of as "God."

In tantra we find happiness by opening our hearts to the people around us, to the world around us, and ultimately to ourselves.

It Is Easier to Love a Theory Than It Is to Love People

The great religious texts—the Bible, the Koran, the Bhagavad Gita, and the Torah—tell us, by metaphor, anecdote, and literal instruction, to love others. Most people with a conscience, religious or otherwise, will agree that love and compassion are among the most noble of ambitions. Why, then, is there so much hatred, war, and misery? Why does the actual practice of love not always coincide with that which is idealized?

To many of us God is a concept. God is known by many different names: Universal Consciousness, Almighty, Energy, Creator, Source, Goddess, Mother-Father God, Yahweh, and Allah, to name a few. God is that part within us that knows we are part of something larger than ourselves, that there is a pattern to this life of ours, and that somehow we are linked to one another. Whatever we may call this source of inspiration, one thing rings clear. How much tangible harm can he/she/it do to us from seemingly far away?

People are quite another matter. People make mistakes, hurt our feelings, disappoint us. It's not easy to love someone who appears to cause us harm. It's not a simple task to let go of the small hurts, intentional and otherwise, that inevitably accumulate over time with family, friends, neighbors, and lovers. We get bruised, and we remember these bruises. We build walls to prevent pain.

Thus, the ideal of love, as espoused by spiritual teachings, becomes very, very challenging. It is easier protect ourselves, to make our love conditional, and to withhold our love with mature and rational logic. After all, as long as we can justify our pain or anger with good reasons, our lack of love, even our malicious deeds toward others, is excusable.

Tantra has no text or manual on how to treat others. Yet the universal call for love within all great spiritual teachings can be embodied through tantra. Tantra calls our intellectual bluff. Tantra takes the theory of loving God to a practical level. Before we can love God, we must love others. Tantra asks us not to idealize love, or to love a concept, but rather to experience love. Tantra is about really loving others, here and now.

This does not mean that we need to have sex with everyone we want to love. Tantra is a tool that teaches us how to love unconditionally, in every area of our lives. Many people misunderstand how tantra relates to sex. Tantra uses sex only as a vehicle. In and of itself, sex is meaningless. Sex is a tool, like the flame of a candle in meditation or the beads used in prayer. No tool will bring us enlightenment unless we use it for that purpose. Tantra's purpose is never about having sex. The purpose of tantra is not even to be tantric. The purpose of tantra is, once again, love. Tantra holds sexuality in a context that is healing and positive, as an expression of God's love. My sexuality was to become a primary channel for strengthening my spiritual life.

People become involved in tantra for various reasons. The practice of tantra can bring us many personal benefits, including improved relationships, emotional healing, physical health, longevity, happiness, wealth, and of course the obvious: an intensely satisfying sex life. I chose tantra for many reasons, some of which I would not discover for many years. But, regardless of diverse initial interests, to remain on this path all must have only one agenda—a profound desire for oneness with whatever it is we call God.

Path of the Heart

Tantra might be a simple path, but it is not always easy. Many people who begin tantra, even with the best intentions, will fall off the path. Why is it so difficult to make love all the time? Practicing tantra is not like going to church for two hours a week. It will make us look at ourselves. It will ask us to change. It pushes buttons. Indeed, it pushed buttons inside me that I didn't know I had.

The methodology of tantra is feminine, which is a striking difference when compared to Western spirituality. Western thought—which has been biased in favor of masculine values for these past two thousand years of patriarchy—values rationality, scientific analysis, and rules. The way of tantra is through the heart. The heart is ruled by love, not logic. Through our hearts, we give and receive of ourselves: not just our intellectual wisdom, but also our empathy, intimacy, and joyful passion. We become the nurturers and providers, as a mother with her child, as Earth with her bounty.

All of us, regardless of gender, have some degree of masculine and feminine characteristics. Through the eyes of tantra, when we bring these aspects of ourselves into balance, we begin to feel more centered: more of a whole person. For example, a woman who is dominated by logic and blind ambition might find tantra strengthening her inner qualities of intuition and compassion. An overly emotional man, on the other hand, will become more rational and in control. It is very possible to have both sides out of balance, as was my predicament. In the case of my outward ambitions, I was independent to the point of being too self-involved. Yet I lacked a strong sense of emotional grounding, which caused me considerable insecurity and self-doubt. I had my work cut out for me!

The promises of tantra were great, and almost unbelievable at times. Tantra allows anyone to experience the ecstatic, heavenly realm that saints through the ages have attempted to describe through poetry and metaphor. It's nearly indescribable, because it's beyond what we can mentally conceive. Utilizing our most primitive, overwhelming desires for sexual encounter, tantra teaches transcendence of all desire. Tantra's ultimate lesson is that all human desire carries at its source the singular desire for God. And even the desire for God is transcended once we understand that we are already there.

This dream, remote to many of us even as a possibility, is a real destiny achievable through tantra. The only question for me was: Do I have the courage, strength, and, most important, the faith to accept such a challenge? Stubborn as I am, the choice seemed obvious.

Initiation 2

n fantasy I knew there would be delights, but this that I now feel is beyond mental comprehension—it is both feeling and sensation. Love laced with heat dances inside me, dancing like the coil of smoke rising from a flame. Oh, this dancing warmth is so very deep, immensely thicker than physical heat, it is like a presence between us that is blessing our long anticipated union. Namaste, I bow to the divinity within you.

It is the eve of my tantric initiation. Just before sunset I enter the tantric home of my teachers. An inviting fireplace warms the living room. The scent of sandalwood incense evokes a memory of church pews. Soft music plays in the background, a mixture of Eastern and Western melody. There is no book here to read, nor rules to follow, nor any sermon to ponder. I feel a gentle peace warming my body and my heart.

There must be lots of sex that goes on within these walls, but how is it that it feels spiritual and pure, like a familiar church? The tantric home—its softness, innocence, and feeling of encompassing love—incites contradictions within me.

As I await my teacher, who is preparing for this initiation as I have already done, my mind begins to wander. Now twenty-one, I consider myself a sexually liberated woman. In my mind, at least. The tantrics I have met so far are quite sexual, whereas until now my imagination has lived a much richer life than has my physical body. Tantrics, as I have noticed, are happy and confident. And radiant! Some of the *tantrikas** I know are twice my age, but they look young enough to be my sisters. How do they maintain such physical youth and vitality? How can they have so much sex, yet appear so innocent?

He enters the room, freshly bathed. Similar to the connection I felt with his wife, I knew immediately that he would be my tantric partner. His wife, herself a beautiful tantric teacher who radiates a vitality I have rarely seen, was perfectly agreeable to this arrangement. It sounds strange, I know. It took me two years to get accustomed to the idea.

We hug. We disrobe. We share a small amount of wine and some cheese and crackers. We talk about what we will do. We talk about our feelings.

"I'm nervous," I confess, blushing.

He asks me, for the hundredth time, if I'm sure I'm ready. He shares that, even as a man, he was once very nervous as well. I ask him how he got over it.

He replies, "I just went beyond my fears and I did it."

Deep inside, I know I'm ready.

We hold hands, and ask for God to join us. My heart beats wildly. And then we begin to breathe in unison.

How very different it feels to breathe in unison so intimately with another person. Our energies, first disconnected and unfocused, begin to integrate in harmony as a singular unit. On completion, we sit in silence, enjoying the vibrant stillness that is our creation. My body's energy has shifted from nervous to peaceful. I feel present.

We sit in the position of *yab-yum*—that is, I sit on his lap, my legs around him, while he sits upright and cross-legged. We breathe as one. On inhale we visualize energy coming up from the earth, in through our root chakra at the perineum,† and up our spine. As we exhale, we send the energy from our

---

*A *tantrika* is a female tantric practitioner.

†The *root chakra* is the energetic equivalent to the perineum, known as the first chakra, where we pull energy into the body (see chapter 3). The *perineum* is the soft spot that sits just between the anus and the sex organs.

hearts into the heart and down the spine to the root chakra of the other.

As we continue this tantric breathing, I feel a strange sense of relief. I'm not sure why or how. I feel a closeness, a deep trust in my partner. I feel a part of myself relaxing that has not relaxed in a long, long time.

A deep crimson fills the room as the final rays of the sunset stroke the western sky. Swollen from desire, I feel I might reach orgasm just from the breathing. I beckon to him for more.

He places himself between my legs and begins to circle his tongue around what he calls my yoni, the gentle tantric word for a woman's sacredness.

I'm so excited that I know I could achieve orgasm at any moment. But he proceeds very, very slowly, taking time to explore every little detail of me. It's different from the way of other men I have been with, who in a rush press on me harder and harder in hopes that I might climax sooner. My tantric partner seems to delight in the actual experience, as though nothing else in the world matters.

For the first time, I stop trying to have an orgasm. I just enjoy him—his tongue's every twist, turn, and tease. As he licks, I breathe. Up through my spine and out my heart, the energy of God flows through me. All thoughts disappear except for this moment of now.

I am so close to orgasm that my legs shake, and then he slows the rhythm of his tongue, letting my excitement abate for a while. Then he increases the pace so that my heart quickens and I come close to orgasm, my legs shaking more than before, and again he backs off. Each time I get more and more aroused, so that finally, after an hour, I am nearly begging him to let me come. Finally I slip over that edge and convulse in the sweetest ecstasy I have ever experienced. I expect him to stop but he doesn't. He continues to arouse me and take me to climax several times more. Each orgasm gets increasingly intense. A tantric man must have a very strong tongue!

He lies down and asks permission to penetrate me.* I smile and slowly bring his lingam† completely inside me. My yoni, wet and aching for him, seeks this completion. Our bodies move in slow rhythm. We are visualizing

---

*In tantric tradition it is customary for a man to ask permission to go inside his partner each time they make love. I find this to be an incredibly respectful and gentlemanly gesture!

†Lingam is the tantric word for a man's penis.

the energy circuit, moving in huge currents now through our aroused sexu-ality, through our spines and out our hearts and down into the other. My whole body climaxes, once, then again, then a third time. I lie on my back and he again enters me. His motions are slow and deliberate, matching my own energy. When he reaches orgasm, he gazes into my eyes in reverence and love.

That night I sleep like a rock in bed with him. The next morning I awaken at sunrise. I feel a warm, thick buzzing in my body, unlike anything I have experienced before. My body feels totally present, yet not in an excited or nervous way. I feel light as air, and at the same time completely grounded. Everything in the world is right. I feel no hunger whatsoever for the entire day.

And that was just the first time.

Essentials 3

ove is my ointment, my lubrication, my wetness that wells from deep inside me. Love keeps the body young, the joints oiled. Love is the tingling up the spine, to the neck, into the head. Love is soft. Love is forever. Love is the sunrise and sunset that continue infinitely. Love is the only constant, the inextinguishable. Love is the beginning, and love will be the end. Love is why I am here.

Until my initiation I had thought that understanding tantra's mysteries required deep analysis and penetrative thought. But it was not my ability to analyze that helped me really embody tantra; it was in the doing. Tantra is a path of action. Now an initiate, it was time for me to put into use the three fundamental requirements of tantric lovemaking: ritual, a partner, and the mutual intention of love.

My partner and I began to practice tantra once a week, first at his tantric home and later, once I moved out of my parents' house and into an apartment, we practiced at mine. These sessions lasted an average of three hours. It was not easy finding this kind of spare time between the demands of college and work. But in tantra, as in every area of life, we gain our greatest results depending on how consistent we are.

In order to establish discipline and consistency, tantra uses ritual. *Ritual* can be defined as repetitive action with a purpose and that causes habit. Through tantra, I would begin to build my habit of experiencing spiritual oneness.

But don't all religions incorporate some kind of ritual? In this sense it was hard for me to understand how tantra diverges from any religion. My teacher was quick to point out that ritual is a lot different from dogma.

Dogma, according to *Webster,* is a "body of doctrines concerning faith or morals formally stated and authoritatively proclaimed by a church."* Dogma tells us what's good and what's bad: it's a framework of morals. All major religions today are based on dogma. Dogma mandates actions. From dogma, religion instructs us what to do and what not to do.

Tantra does not require belief in dogma; thus, there is no ordained behavior either to follow or to avoid. There is not even a system of philosophy. But what about the many books I had read about tantra? Surely most tantric teachers have strong opinions. Naturally, we do not live inside a vacuum, so most tantric teachers integrate the unique customs and beliefs that are influenced by their culture and religion. I found that some of the teachings even contradict each other.

Because there are no rules in tantra, this is not a path for the weak. Weak people want structure. Instead, tantra brings with it personal power and freedom. This does not mean rebellion or anarchy. What we learn through tantra is internal. It challenges every fear-based limitation that we have inside ourselves.

But I did find that tantra does tend to call into question conventional social customs and behaviors that are often based on dogma. In India, a country whose religion was predominantly Hinduism, tantric ritual used elements that were specifically forbidden by that religion. These are the five *makaras,* and they include meat, ritualistic sex, and even a mild aphrodisiac (similar to wine).

Instead of blindly obeying the established order and conventional thought, we can listen to the voice of truth within. Dogma becomes our individual choice.

Webster's Ninth New Collegiate Dictionary (Springfield, Mass.: Merriam-Webster, 1985): 373.

Thus, I realized, tantra cannot be a religion, nor does it inherently conflict with religion. Tantra is forever new and fluid, just as we must be. Every spiritual path comes from inside each person and is as unique as each individual.

In the abstract sense, ritual is irrelevant to the practice of tantra. Along those lines, even sexual intercourse is not necessary. But this is like saying that an Olympic athlete need not train because she already has the potential to win. In practicality, the path of tantra is quite ritualistic. And very sexual.

Tantra is a fluid methodology that becomes actuated within ritual. Human beings intrinsically resist change. Tantra, being all about change—change that can be extremely fast—uses the comfortable context of habit to help us grow and evolve. We use tantric ritual to develop the habit of letting go of our fear more quickly.

The most important component of ritual is purpose, or intention. Without a purpose, the most beautiful and elaborate ritual will be wasted. In tantra the ultimate purpose is to become one with ourselves, with others, and with whatever we define as God. During tantric lovemaking we honor God by lovingly worshiping our partner. The tantric form of partner worship does not replace the worship of God—we are merely experiencing the aspect of our partner that is pure divinity or perfection. We are seeing his or her highest potential. The concepts of oneness with God, or love, or absolute consciousness, become embodied: I can viscerally touch and feel and know, beyond the perception of my limited mind, what these things mean.

Ritual includes all the practices and methodologies that are part of tantric lovemaking. Some of these rituals I learned in advance, but most I discovered in the actual doing. I had learned about the sexual *asanas* (positions) such as the *yab-yum, indrani,* and *kakila*. I had learned about the energy circuits and where to focus my mind's eye. But most of the meditations and practices came to me spontaneously. Even though my partner was a tantric teacher with many years of experience, I actually initiated most of the meditations that we did.

One day I asked my partner's wife about this. She was a beautiful and powerful tantrika in her own right and emanated a sweetness the likes of which I have rarely seen.

"You are guiding the process because you are the woman," she said. "A woman is more inherently capable of intuiting the right things to do during tantric lovemaking."

The Need for Another

Tantra is well regarded within the yoga tradition as the fastest path to enlightenment. Eastern legend holds that an average human soul takes 100,000 lifetimes to achieve enlightenment, but that with tantra, any person truly committed to this path can gain enlightenment in as little as one lifetime. I soon discovered why this is true.

It has to do with the amount of energy available to us. During tantra we are able to use both our own energy and that of our partner. The total energy produced is much greater than the sum of its parts. Energy incites change. The more energy we have, the faster the rate of change. When we combine the energy of two people toward a common purpose, spiritual development accelerates at an exponential rate.

Many students of God acknowledge a teacher who serves as their inspiration in this physical world. To Hasidic Jews this person is the rebbe. In Catholicism it is a priest or the pope. Your tantric partner will become your teacher and you will become his. Some partners are at the same level of conscious spiritual evolvement. Sometimes there is one dominant teacher. My partner had a far greater level of emotional evolvement than I, and he was also much better at containing and directing tantric energy. For the most part I consider him my teacher, even though in tantric practice I was initiating the various positions and meditations. But sometimes I would teach him some things. (You cannot teach without learning, they say.) It was touching to me that this strong, accomplished tantric teacher could also be so vulnerable. It made him more approachable to me.

Tantric partners share such a strong bond that in some ways they become very dependent on each other. This might seem a contradiction to the concept of personal responsibility. But mutual dependence does not mean giving up control of our lives. It actually means the opposite; it means each of you takes responsibility for the other. It means letting our partners into our hearts. We do not give up anything; we add to what we already have.

Within a tantric partnership, each person becomes reliant on the sexual and spiritual skills of the other. Our partners must be capable of great empathy and oneness, so that they can understand our emotional, physical, and spiritual rhythms. Furthermore, our partners must understand us so deeply that they know our potential, the perfection of what we can become. Paramount is the need for another.

The need for another. As much as I enjoyed my tantric partner's company and respected his knowledge and experience, I did not like the idea of relying on anyone at all. My independence set me apart. It made me who I am. An individualist! A pioneer! A lover of personal freedom. Autonomy was my sole comfort zone. Yet to follow a path of tantra, I—prodigal loner— must choose to rely on someone else for my personal spiritual pursuits.

Well, that's inconvenient, I grumbled to myself. After all, my spiritual path is between God and me. Why bother depending on someone? It would be a lot easier just to take this information and use it by myself. I had it in the back of my mind that I could do tantra differently. Sure, tantra requires a partner, *except in my case, that is.* I'm told that this is a common feeling with new students. But could I get over it?

There is no place within the human spirit more vulnerable than the heart. The heart is where we feel the deepest pain. We summon our greatest strength from the heart. In tantra the hardest step—allowing another person into the heart in deep trust and oneness—will bring the greatest reward.

When I looked more deeply at my aversion to this idea, I realized it was not my independence or freedom I was afraid of losing: I was afraid of being hurt by others. A protective wall covering my heart kept me safe. Defensiveness was my armor against pain. Any child raised in an unhappy family knows what hurt is all about. We learn that relationships are painful, that they lead to separation even when we have the best of intentions.

My earliest memories of relationships were of struggle and sorrow. Brothers betraying my trust, sisters rejecting me, a mother in too much pain to pay me enough attention, a father not understanding. As a sensitive child, I took all of this deeply to heart, and as an adult I was still not eager to show my vulnerability. So much of my past was unconsciously running my life.

Ultimately, my fear of being hurt had nothing to do with anyone outside of me. It had nothing to do with siblings, parents, or friends. I was weighed down by painful memories as though they were stronger than I. But, in fact, the protective barriers I placed in front of my heart kept me from experiencing love. The walls did not protect me; they prevented me from knowing who I am. They kept me from giving and receiving the love and joy my true nature yearned for.

The heart is so vast! How are we to contain such a wild part of ourselves? My heart was a place within my soul that I didn't really know, and I feared it was something I couldn't control. I was afraid that if I really let myself open up to someone, logic would fly out the window and I would become a victim of enormous, overpowering waves of love. I would be unable to protect myself if the need arose. I would be unable to set personal boundaries. I would turn into a big pile of mushy love with no backbone.

Yet did my fear make sense? Why would I not be able to control my heart? Why would that be beyond me? After all, my heart is within me.

The Intention of Love

Within each of us there is a longing that transcends the boundaries of our bodies and emotions. This need is the shadow of remembrance—we are part of something larger than ourselves. We come from somewhere. There is a higher purpose to our lives. Known also as oneness with the divine cosmos or human enlightenment, we seek to fill this innate yearning through religion, art, and science.

The great barrier to our embodiment of this source is misperception. Vedic philosophy calls it *maya*, or the misperception that this temporal world is our true reality. In Buddhism, believing in the illusion (that we are separate from the source) results in *dukkha,* or suffering. Christian religion has given it a personality: the devil, the angel who fell from God's grace, who is living apart from God. Modern psychology calls it fear. Fear stands for False Evidence Appearing Real. When we fear, we feel lack; we are separate from the source and need to find it.

Many times my teacher would say that the goal of tantra is oneness with self, others, and God. But what does "oneness" mean? I never really understood oneness until I started feeling it at an emotional level.

My first experience of oneness was through complete acceptance. For example, when I am at one with my fear of trusting others, then I can nurture and love this part of me instead of fighting or repressing the fear. I am neither condoning nor judging myself. I am merely being. It is not that I want to continue to distrust. But I won't be able to change anything until I'm one with my fear. I learned to be conscious and in the moment, with no judgment and no preconceived ideas about what should be.

Oneness in the context of relationships means accepting people as they are, without wanting them to be different. It means letting go of expectations and viewing their personalities or actions as neither superior nor inferior. It means simply knowing people as they are, and accepting them in totality.

People are our mirrors. We love or hate people because of what we respectively admire or despise in ourselves. If I can accept another person, I am ultimately accepting myself.

Oneness was really hard for me. It took a lot of practice because I had always been extremely self-critical. I expected to live up to a fantasy of perfection I had in my mind. I had to be thin, beautiful, successful, wealthy, and loved by everyone. I was so hard on myself. Compared to any wrong that anyone had ever done to me, I hurt myself a hundred times more, just because I was so self-judging.

This tendency spilled into my relationships, of course. I demanded perfection in others. I put people on pedestals and inevitably they came crashing down.

In tantra I would learn to change this habit through accepting just one person in totality. Just one! As I learned to do this during the act of tantra, an amazing thing happened. All of my relationships started to change. I began to learn how to accept my friends and family.

"You are really growing up," I heard others telling me.

The same effect happens during meditation. In meditation we silence our minds' chatter for perhaps thirty minutes per day, but the effect on the rest of our lives is significant, for we begin to feel more peaceful and calm. In sports we might spend only a few hours a week training, but the results are overall health, energy, and mental clarity.

Oneness is not instantaneous. I did not just decide to be one and then everything sort of fell into place. It took consistent effort. Still, I somehow thought that I should be "getting" this lesson faster than I was.

"How long do I need to work on this?" I asked. "I think I'm doing pretty well here. People are even commenting on my changes!"

"Valerie, my impatient one," said my teacher, laughing, "you have just begun. Oneness can easily take a lifetime to master."

But wouldn't Prozac be much easier?

Spiritual Oneness

I began to realize that oneness is not one-dimensional. There are many subleties to this form of art that I was learning through tantra. The next step would bring me even more happiness! Now I was really getting into the fun part of tantra.

Spiritual oneness goes beyond who and what we think we are—the aspects that make up our personalities. It goes beyond acceptance and compassion. Spiritual oneness brings God into our experience of acceptance. Spiritual oneness occurs when we are attuned to another's spirit. We experience the divinity or essence of others. We are beyond seeing their personalities or their interactions with us, be they good or bad. We see only what is true: only what lies within the deepest core of their hearts. We see the God within them.

Spiritual oneness is always accompanied by deep love, for to see into the essence of another is to see perfection.

Spiritual oneness is the opposite of expectations. The reason that we have expectations is because we care. We should not stop caring; we should merely transform our expectations from wanting another to behave as we desire into seeing what is his highest potential, perhaps even beyond what he himself knows. We see a partner as a physical embodiment of divine love. A tantric teacher once defined tantra to me as the act of making love with the mind-set that we are the God and Goddess in passionate embrace.

When we tap into a person's divinity, we are able to guide him to seeing that perfection within himself. We become the teacher, like a coach who sees the potential of a great athlete. We can physically train his body to encompass more joy, which is his true nature. We can hold the space for his emotional misperceptions to surface and be healed. We can hold the intention and prayer in our minds for his own spiritual awakening.

Spiritual oneness begins during tantra with our physical senses, such as sight, touch, and taste. These senses, which normally perceive the subjective world that lies within the confines of our skin and mind, now expand outward, to our partners. *We teach our senses to go inside our partners.* Once attuned to my partner's physical self, I can open my heart and feel his emotions. I can feel what might be upsetting him and silently send energy and love into his pain. I can rejoice in his pleasure so that I hold the space for his happiness. I use my mind's eye to see his spiritual vision.*

The experience of spiritual oneness during tantra really began to affect my interpretation of God. It's as if during tantra there's more happening than just the experience of myself and my partner. It seems as though there are three present: myself, my partner, and a residing energy that I cannot describe except that it seems like God. This energy feels warm and thick and comforting, residing both within and outside my body. It blurs the line between myself and my partner. When we achieve spiritual oneness during tantric lovemaking, this too will affect our daily lives.

I began to regain the highly developed sense of intuition I had as a young child. As a little girl I had a "psychic" gift of knowing precisely what others were feeling and why. I could actually read their emotional states. Quite early in life I had buried this ability. It was just too painful to feel the hurt of others. Now I have remembered this skill, but as an adult I know how to manage my feelings so that I can help others without hurting myself. This ability to be one with another's emotions positively affects both my personal and professional relationships. It helps me go beyond the words that people are saying and know what they really feel and need.

The three simple requirements of tantra—ritual, a partner, and the mutual intention of love—brought up my fears, self-imposed barriers, and hidden agendas. I was full of pain and confusion. Despite my resistance I kept going, because everything in my life was getting better. Tantra was working wonders. At times I would marvel at all that I was learning in such a short period. And there was much, much more to come.

*The third eye, a chakra located at the center of the forehead, is known as the spiritual eye.

Chakras and Kundalini

I am seeing planes of sensory experience that I never new could exist! These planes travel deeper into the essence of me, transcending time and space—yet I have no fear. My true self is blossoming. Not by direction or force, just by surrender. And now my sexuality and heart are becoming so merged that I can hardly put my attention on one without exciting the other. So ecstatic that I begged he return tomorrow.

A warm buzzing up my spine, a glowing light inside my head, a gentle glow within my heart tightening in my stomach, a tickling constriction in my throat—these were the manifestations of the esoteric concepts within Eastern literature that I had so often questioned. Some sensations came upon me during the first few weeks of tantra; others took years. But one thing was certain: I was beginning to see the world around me differently, beyond my eyes' perceptions.

Chakras

Chakras, meaning "wheels" or "circles," are the centers of highest energy in the body. Chakras cannot be seen with the physical eye. However, in auric photography, in which chakras have actually been captured on film, they appear as wheels of energy surrounding the body. Chakras are part of us, affecting us just as do our legs and arms.

Chakras work in conjunction with the physical state and can be used in tantra to cleanse the body, to build energy, and to induce positive emotional states. The body has seven main chakras, each corresponding to a specific emotion, as well as to a particular area of the body.

Chakra	Body Area	Characteristic
Root	Perineum	Survival/aliveness
Sex	Sex organs	Sexual desire
Power	Stomach	Strength/willpower
Heart	Heart	Love
Throat	Throat	Truth and integrity
Third eye	Middle of forehead	Intuition
Crown	Top of head	Spiritual insight

Chakras can act as indicators of our feelings even before we're consciously aware of the feelings. If we are off balance or upset, the energy of tantra will bring forth certain feelings that seem to emanate from a particular chakra. If my throat feels tight and constricted, perhaps it's because I am not fully expressing myself. If my heart is hurting, I may be withholding love.

During tantra, sensations within the chakras will become intensified. Tantra's momentum of energy will bring forth any feelings that may be lying dormant within our chakras. The tantric process has the very beneficial effect of getting us "out of our heads" and into the present moment. Be prepared to know thyself! Experiencing the multiple levels of chakras and their subtleties is a blessing to anyone who overanalyzes like me. My habit of judging the past and worrying about the future was about to be changed forever.

The mind is our greatest asset, but without discipline it can easily pull us out of the present moment and condemn us to a world of mind chatter. The physical body, however, is always present. When we are attuned to our body, our mind also becomes present.

Chakras can teach us much about ourselves. Paying attention to our chakras helps us know exactly what we're feeling. The advice to "Follow your heart" and the phrase *gut instinct* began to take on whole new meanings.

But this was not just a passive exercise. I learned how to use my chakras to change my emotional state. If, for example, I want to forgive someone, during tantra I focus my mind on my heart chakra. I can see my heart opening and expanding, letting go of any constriction or pain. Energy is a great cleansing agent. It helps us let go of all kinds of emotional baggage very quickly.

Kundalini

A spiritual person displays certain characteristics, such as compassion, selflessness, and a forgiving nature. But the spiritual self does not evolve in a vacuum. Every part of us is interconnected. The physical body is also capable of spiritual evolvement. When this happens, it too begins to emanate certain characteristics. These characteristics are the result of what is called kundalini.

Kundalini has been referenced in nearly all major spiritual teachings by different names, both obscurely and specifically. It has been called spiritual elixir, divine nectar, the sleeping serpent, a manifestation of the Holy Spirit, and the light of God.

Kundalini can be either dormant (sleeping) or active (awakened). It is felt inside the body as a very specific type of energy. In most people, kundalini is dormant. In its inactive state we feel nothing of its presence.

But what a tremendous potential is the kundalini! When through the practice of tantra we awaken this potential within us, the kundalini uncoils itself like a serpent, starting from the base of the spine, in the region of the coccyx. Tremendous energies rise up the spine and spread throughout the body. Anyone who has achieved enlightenment has awakened this kundalini.

Through various techniques, we first charge the energy that sits at the base of the spine. At some point this energy will become activated and begin to flow up the spine. The energy rises up the *sushumna,* the central canal located in the spine, through each chakra, into the top of the head, stimulating areas within the brain and outward, mixing with the energy of universal consciousness. Thus fused, the energy then journeys back down the spine through the root chakra. The energy has balance. When it flows upward it is a cool blue, female in nature, also known as lunar energy. When it flows downward, it is hot and feels like an orange-red energy.

Kundalini opens up energies and cleanses all the chakras, starting from the root chakra, located at the perineum. From there, each chakra higher will become enlivened, continuing upward and outward to the crown chakra, located at the top of the head, lighting up dormant parts of the mind and spirit.

Kundalini is the body's way of connecting us to our higher self. The entire process of awakening kundalini usually takes many years. Once kundalini is awakened, there is no turning it off. The stages of kundalini awakening vary widely, from imperceptible changes that hardly affect us to complete, dramatic shifts that require years of adjustment. We always want kundalini to awaken slowly and gradually, never all at once.

It has not been documented medically exactly how kundalini changes the body's physiology, but one thing is certain: it strongly affects the spinal cord and the entire nervous system. It feels like an electrical current coursing through the body, cleansing and energizing it. Kundalini can have a life of its own. It has a wisdom that is beyond our logical mind. Because of this, it can be difficult to control kundalini beyond simply limiting the amount of tantra we practice.

Tantra has a clear advantage over other forms of yoga in awakening kundalini because of the access to sexual energy. However, we must be cautious about awakening kundalini through tantra. Before attempting to do so, I was instructed to learn other breathing practices and disciplines that would prepare my body. Some of my favorites were stretching and breathing exercises.

In order to loosen up and awaken the spine, we would do several spine stretches. These included standing up and bending at the waist, arms relaxed, to elongate the spine (exhaling on the way down and inhaling on the way back up). Then we would do slow twists from the waist while standing upright (exhaling on the twist and inhaling on return to center). Then we would lie on the floor, on our stomachs, and, using our arms, stretch the upper body upward while leaving the pelvis area touching the floor. Then we would come down and lift our hips in the air so that the body formed an inverted V. I learned many stretching exercises like this that really charged my body with energy.

We also did a great deal of breathing exercises. To get the feel of energy flowing up the body, upon inhale we visualize energy coming up the spine starting from the perineum and up to the crown chakra, and upon exhale we visualize it going back down the front of the body. Then we would meditate on each individual chakra for several minutes each, by pulling energy directly into the chakra upon inhale and seeing the chakra fill with light. Then we exhaled.

Disciplining the mind, however, is the most important aspect of preparing for the kundalini awakening. Without proper preparation, kundalini can be painful. *Just as kundalini will increase positive characteristics within us, it will also very quickly amplify every negative tendency we have.* Its purpose is to cleanse us. It works like a sculptor, who starts with a block of clay and keeps chipping away the debris until all that remains is the art itself. I have heard of people going nearly insane from the energy because they were not prepared for it. I, too, struggled through some very rough times, both emotionally and physiologically (see chapter 10).

During tantra the energy we generate that activates our kundalini and chakras will make our bodies become superbly intelligent because they align the body with the spirit, or higher self. Because emotions are stored in the body, emotional healing can happen very quickly through tantra. An issue that could take years to overcome in traditional psychotherapy may be resolved in days, or even moments, when kundalini is present.

But of themselves, these physiological awakenings do not mean that we become emotionally and spiritually enlightened by default; they merely speed up the process. There is no such thing as a spiritual shortcut. Simultaneous to any kundalini awakening we must constantly train our emotions and minds to contain the evolvement of our bodies.*

---

*For more information about kundalini, I highly recommend *Kundalini* by Gopi Krishna (Shambhala Publications, 1967).

Some theories suggest that kundalini cannot be activated by merely our will alone. This spiritual gift requires both our intense desire and a blessing by God, as though God holds the key to this energy and will allow for its unlocking only when we are ready. Ultimately, though, any spiritual insight or growth involves our relationship to source, and kundalini is no different.

The arousal of kundalini is not the purpose of tantra. The purpose of tantra never stops at its physical ramifications: neither blissful sex nor a full kundalini awakening is the destination. The arousal of kundalini energy is simply a tool by which the sustaining purpose of tantra—enlightenment and oneness with God—is achieved.

On beginning tantric practice I found that one effective method of stimulating kundalini is through oral sex. My partner and I practiced both in a closed circuit (commonly known as 69), giving oral pleasure at the same time to each other, and one at a time, where one person gives and the other lies back and receives. The energy circuit allows the energy to flow up our spines, out our tongues, and directly into the root and sex chakras of our partners, which are precisely where the kundalini energy first gets released. From there our partners can take the energy and pull it up into the spine, through the chakras, into the brain and outward.

The advantage of the closed circuit is that the energy flows bidirectionally, so there is more energy to work with. In the beginning, however, it is easier to concentrate if we practice one person at a time.

During oral pleasuring I often feel huge currents of kundalini charging from my coccyx and up into my spine, right at orgasm. It feels almost like a miniature explosion inside my coccyx, like a warm sac filled with fluid bursting open and pouring out and upward.

Most of the time, kundalini feels like an internal massage that gently lubricates my body. The first time I felt it was two years into practicing tantra, at the age of twenty-three. I awoke in the morning and felt a cool blue light flowing from my coccyx upward into my spine and up to the base of my neck. At first, groggy from the night before, I thought I may have spilled water on the bed. I got up but my back was dry. It didn't hurt; in fact, it felt calming and peaceful. It felt like both cold and hot energy flowing from the base of my spine—the coccyx, upward through my spine, into my head.

At first the energy was centralized in my spine. Over time it began to spread outward through my back, up my head, down my arms and legs. Eventually it came around to the front of my body, and now it settles frequently in one or more chakras at any given time. The energy has become more normal and more comfortable. It changes patterns often. This moment as I am writing, I feel its cool blue presence as energy in my upper back, between my shoulder blades, and up into the front of my neck, and it gets cooler as it flows upward into my head. It feels as if there is a sweet, nectarlike substance flowing just inside my skin. I feel its presence almost all the time—even at night.

The first few years I practiced tantra, and now on occasion, I got what is known as the sweats. This is when you perspire profusely during the night because of the intense internal heat that the kundalini generates. The strongest kundalini adjustments or awakenings seem to occur when the body is at rest, during the body's parasympathetic phase. Kundalini thus feels quite strong in the early morning, just before bed, and during and after tantra or meditation. It can also feel intense when I am concentrating intently.

Most of the time kundalini makes me feel utterly blissful. But it can be strange; I would feel all these blissful things going on in my body, as though my body were singing or laughing, but everything around me was exactly the same. At school I would want to share this feeling that made me want to laugh with joy. But how could I explain this phenomenon to others? How could I share the ecstasy? Sometimes this depressed me, because I wanted to bring the happiness with me into the world so that others could feel it also. Sometimes I felt isolated and alone as I went through the day.

Once awakened, kundalini causes an intensely heightened conscience. It clashes with anything negative in the body: anger, fear, lack of faith, distrust, harmful agendas. It naturally causes us to gravitate to better characteristics, such as generosity, compassion, gratitude, and forgiveness. This is understandable—it is the reflection of our true nature.

Kundalini is the guru inside us. It would not surprise me if the concept of hell originated from the internal hell a person's body can go through if he is not living in integrity with love and compassion. I went through a bit of internal hell as I learned to adjust my self-serving values to the values of my higher self.

Kundalini seems to shine light into the dark sides of our personalities, and that's when we experience physical pain. The energy of kundalini appears to collide with anything negative in its path. When I was doing something that was not in my best interest, or spending time with someone who was not good for me, I would feel it in my body. Depending on the issue, I would feel the pain as nausea (power chakra), heartburn (heart chakra), or a headache (third eye chakra).

As stubborn as I can be, I did learn relatively quickly how to manage this resistance, because kundalini takes no prisoners. Either you learn to face your resistance, or you are in pain. And indeed, there was much, much resistance that I would face.

Ritual 5

I am hypnotized by the rhythmic music—the ruby red of my sheets matches the blood that my yoni is engorged with, even hours afterward. This sacred space we create enhances the mood. It heats up my body, and I feel like I am in a trance. I can close my eyes and a blissful, dreamlike state washes over me—not sleeping, not awake. I feel sexual, powerful, erotic, alive, so grounded and heavenly at the same time. I forget all my problems and flaws and dive into this idyllic dream of sweat and wetness that is too good to believe.

Every woman wants to feel special. And how very special tantric ritual made me feel: like the most beautiful woman on Earth, like my happiness was the sole concern of the universe, like I was supported and loved in every way.

"Don't worry," teased my partner so many times, "it gets better."

Tantric ritual has been influenced by many factors—social customs, cultural heritage, and religion, for example. This forever-evolving art form honors our individuality while embracing a vast legacy. Ritual is both personal and richly communal. We can read many books about tantric ritual. But we can also listen to the moon and the waters and the wind and, above all, our hearts.

Through tantric ritual we establish practices that we do not normally perform during traditional sex. This prepares us to know that something very special is in store.

Ritual should be simple, especially for people like me who are seduced by the siren of complication. When my partner and I set out to create our own ritual, we wanted just enough to establish a sense of sacredness and an awareness that God is present with us.

Maithuna

Maithuna—meaning "sexual union"—is the fancy word for the daily practice of tantric lovemaking. *Jewel in the Lotus* says of the maithuna: "if the ritual is successful it is possible to achieve enlightenment in a single practice."* Maithuna involves two people, generally you and your mate or tantric partner.† The maithuna is a daily affirmation of the spiritual purpose of the relationship, or active expression of the relationship. (The worshiping of the female principle is done in a compellingly different way, but more on that later.)

A pleasant and sultry atmosphere is created through incense, candles, music. This atmosphere should be consistent. If incense is used, that same incense should be used continuously. Both parties wash themselves. They share a meal consisting of a small amount of meat, fish, grain, and wine. Then parts of the woman's body are anointed with oil, mantras are repeated, and the man excites the woman through foreplay. Once the woman is aroused, the man enters her, and they continue to make love in a very deliberate pattern. At all times it is essential to be clearly aware of the divinity of one's partner and of the sacredness of this act. During this lovemaking the couple focus on the energy circuit between them and direct the energy consciously. Intercourse is controlled and little movement occurs. Maithuna should be performed daily. It generally lasts an hour, but if it is not practiced on a daily basis, we extend the experience for two to four hours.

In maithuna, both partners are acutely conscious of the divinity of each other. They have cast aside their daily arguments or problems and are dedi-

---

*Sunyata Saraswati and Bodhi Avinasha, *Jewel in the Lotus* (San Francisco: Kriya Jyoti Tantra Society, 1987): 179.

†In some groups it was customary for a third guru to be present, but not directly participate, acting as a spiritual presence.

cating this hour to honoring the divinity of their relationship.

The second powerful element of maithuna is the conscious focus on the energy circuit. This energy is what will really transform our consciousness. Of no small consequence is the powerful effect it will have on awakening kundalini. In normal solitary meditation, physically speaking we have only our own energy to draw from and to use in order to transform our consciousness. In maithuna we have two additional resources of physical energy: the energy from our loved one and the energy that is created from the both of us (as the whole is always greater than the sum of its parts).

Mental Preparation

My favorite meditation to prepare for tantric ritual is the flame meditation. I sit cross-legged on my bed, without clothing. I bring my attention to my third eye, about an inch in front of my forehead. I visualize the flame of a candle. I see it flicker, a gentle yellow glow, softly darkening toward the center to form a cool blue at its base. It encompasses a shaft of wick, holding on so gently. The flame dances. I hear its soft hissing and crackle as it licks the wax and burns ever so slowly. I let my mind become absorbed into the life of this flame. In so doing, all other thoughts dissipate and I am becoming a clear channel. Then the flame disappears, and I'm conscious of nothing. In nothingness, I find perfect stillness.

Physical Preparation

Once my mind has reached a state of calm I begin my ritual by bathing, to prepare my temple for a lavish feast. Who knows what parts of my temple will be feasted on today? It is best to be prepared for any kind of pleasure. I wash away the clinging worries of the day. I slowly lather rich, vanilla-scented soap over my body. I run my hands over my shoulders and arms, down my breasts, and onto my stomach, experiencing this temple that is mine. I admire my curves and uniqueness. I work my way onto my yoni and anus, placing special attention here on the seat of both sexuality and life. The yoni is truly sacred, to be worshiped for its ability to bring forth life, as much as for its ability to pleasure and to be pleasured.

The anus is a place of mystery, where we release everything in our bodies that does not serve us. The anus holds within it the potential for great pleasure and orgasmic delight. I clean myself thoroughly, in anticipation of what will come. Down my thighs, legs, and feet I wash tenderly and lovingly. I let the water gently rinse away the suds.

Shaving the head, a highly regarded spiritual practice in some Eastern traditions, is said to purify the spirit. In tantra it is nice to know that we do not need to shave our heads. But women can shave other things.

For tantrikas, shaving the yoni in its entirety is a common practice. A shaved, smooth yoni can bring considerable pleasure to one's partner, especially during oral sex. Its splendor unhidden, he can see and taste all of its subtle curves and folds. A shaved yoni is intensely more receptive. It increases sensitivity a hundredfold not only during lovemaking, but at all other times as well.

For all my sisters out there, if you ever want to feel really alive and powerful, try this: Shave completely, then go through your day wearing nothing but a soft and flowing dress. Be sure to take a leisurely walk outside. Let the wind get to know you. Tantrics have long known that women can be having orgasms at all times.

Because the man's lingam has the pleasure of being exposed naturally, he need not shave. However, he should shave his face carefully just before tantra so that no stubble is felt by the woman's delicate skin. The yoni becomes so sensitized during tantra that even the slightest bristly touch can be agonizing. When the ritual of shaving the yoni and the man's face is complete, the skin can communicate in silent, ecstatic oneness.

Once bathed, I slowly dry my body with a thick, luxurious towel. Sometimes I'll put on a sexy silk robe or a translucent dress. Sometimes I approach my partner wearing nothing but a big smile.

Environment

We light two or three scented candles. The flame represents spiritual surrender. It means relinquishing fear, anger, negative memories and emotions: everything that does not serve our best interest. On occasion I will burn sandalwood incense. I dim the lights so the room has a soft, warm glow.

Music

Sound is a powerful tool for meditation. I have a small library of music that I play only during tantric lovemaking. I play one CD during each session. I put my stereo on automatic repeat so that the music will play over and over, for hours on end. I set the volume quite low, so that it doesn't distract from the rhythms that I create with my partner. I have spent much effort trying to find tantric music. Tantric music should pulsate to a slow, earthy beat. It should not overpower or be too exhilarating.

My partner has told me that he uses the music to establish rhythm and a sense of time (in meditation, this can be helpful because we so often lose track of time). Sometimes he uses a 1:1 rhythm, but not always. Sometimes he uses 1:4 or even 1:8. This is why a slow, earthy beat is so important. He normally does not bring me to my first orgasm until the CD has played through one time and is back to the first track.

This is also why it is important to stay with the same music. It allows the body to merge with sound and enables the body to associate that music with tantric ecstasy every time that piece is heard. The music becomes an association for extreme bliss. I am unable to listen to our tantric music now without going into an orbit of ecstasy—this level of intensity gives a whole new meaning to the saying "They're playing our song."

Food

We share a light meal to honor the abundance of Mother Earth. This might be succulent fruit, imported cheese, a small amount of meat, or some home-made soup with bread. We acknowledge our health and the small miracle that is our taste buds. We savor one small glass of good red wine, the tantric drink: its deep burgundy is the color of life flowing through our veins and of Earth's crimson hues. As we toast, we honor the blessing of being alive.

Sharing

We focus on our relationship. We make our partner's words and feelings the most important thing in the world. Sometimes we share what it is we want to experience during tantra.

If we're upset or distracted by problems of the day, we get them off our chest and let them go. We support each other. We do not argue or blame. We simply communicate so that we can end the past and be in the present moment.

Oneness between us is, of course, the ultimate purpose of our tantra this day. Perhaps my partner wants to have less fear and to strengthen his self-confidence, because negative emotions are the reflection of separation. We talk about this from the heart, gently sharing our truth. We do not strategize how we will become one, or how we will let go of fear—tantra will take care of that. Having the intention for this few moments of sharing is enough.

What is most important is to feel the love we have for our partner. We want what is for his or her highest good. Nothing else matters right now

The Prayer for God

We thoughtfully and willfully bring divine grace into our consciousness. Sometimes we pray together. Sometimes we silently gaze into each other's eyes, seeing the God within. We ask God to be with us, that we may feel more oneness and more love, and to help us let go of everything within that desires separation.

Consistency

Historically, the moon has played an important role in the lives of tantrics. As a symbol of feminine energy and power, its unfailing cycles predictably affect all earthly life, from the ocean's changing tides to a woman's menses. Tantra so closely connects us with the rhythms of Earth that the more tantra we do, the closer we feel to the cycles of the Moon.

Some tantric groups have followed the twenty-eight-day lunar cycle, whose calendar is based on the phases of the Moon. There is a lot of folklore about why this is so. One idea comes from the harvest. Farmers typically plant seeds on the new moon and harvest on the full moon; for some reason Mother Nature likes to grow that way. This means that the farm family is busy working during the new moon, and thus has less time for play (or lovemaking). The basic idea is that the more tantric lovemaking we have, the less food we eat and the less work we do. Conversely, at times when we are working intensive and long hours, we are eating more and having sex less.* Also, the infertile portion of a woman's menstrual cycle normally occurs during the full moon: generally the time when women are most sexually aroused and during which pregnancy is not possible. This cycle is akin to the rhythm method of birth control.

During the new moon, we do not practice any tantra for several days. On the day of the full moon, as well as two or three days prior, we practice tantra twice a day, or make them very long sessions (four to six delicious hours).† Between the new and full moon, we continue to practice tantra consistently in a moderate amount, once daily but, of course, those of us living in the real world cannot skip work or school because a full moon requires us to make love all day long.

To satisfy my insatiable curiosity about this moon thing, I decided to spend nine months practicing tantra according to the lunar cycle. I was surprised that this Moon of ours, sitting quietly in the sky, so strongly affected me. For one thing, it was much easier for me to get in the mood to practice tantra. Believe it or not, sexual ecstasy is not an easy discipline. Like any serious undertaking, it can be difficult to maintain the consistent will to practice. I had a lot going on in my life. I had to be disciplined about school, work, theater rehearsal, and also tantra. But following the Moon's cycles made the discipline of tantra somehow seem easier. In essence, I felt that I was not fighting my own patterns. I found that the Moon's patterns were a reflection of my own inner clock.

Our full-moon "marathon tantra," as we like to call it, was mind blowing, to say the least. There have been many occasions, after engaging in six hours of tantric lovemaking, when I found it impossible to walk—not from pain or being sore; quite the opposite. My body was simply afloat in an ocean of sexual energy and I was so sensitized that closing my legs would bring my

---

*Gavin and Yvonne Frost, *Tantric Yoga* (York Beach, Maine: Samuel Weiser, 1989): chapter 6.
†The full moon is traditionally when the tantric ritual known as the *chakra puja* takes place (see chapter 15).

whole body to orgasm. I really could not close my legs!

Not bad for a day's labor.

Eventually, my partner and I settled into a routine that combined both systems. We do tantra per the "normal" calendar and work week at all times during the month—typically three or four days a week for two or three hours each session. At the time of the full moon, we will practice tantra for a long and lovely length of time.

But even practicing tantra once a week will be tremendously beneficial. The moon aspect is secondary; the significant thing is—as always—the intention of love.

The most important rhythm that I learned to follow was my own. Sometimes I would push myself too much, extremist that I am, and the result was that I would turn off to the whole thing and not practice for a month or two. Most of this had to with my fear. I was doing too much too soon. I eventually learned to respect my own boundaries, and instead of burying my head in the sand, I learned consciously to choose: "I will not practice tantra for one month."

Tantra generates a tremendous amount of energy, and often, the more negative parts of us must play catch-up with our physical bodies, which are being, in a sense, made anew. We must give ourselves plenty of time to adjust to the effects of the tantra. Even the most impatient of us will find that the results of tantra occur quickly and with great intensity.

I have known many people who began this path with the best of intentions, saw amazing results, and then practiced so excessively that they hit too many walls at once and then went to the opposite extreme and stopped practicing tantra forever. As I learned, it's better to go slowly. The tantric path requires not just consistent discipline, but also balance.

Tantric Lovers 6

*H*e is opening my entire sexuality, even inches down my inner thighs. His first lick always makes me pulsate just from the anticipation of this pleasure: his attention to every single spot, every sacred piece of flesh! His tongue goes into these circular movements that my body just sings from—movements I cannot replicate, they seem like heavenly patterns that no one but he knows. I am becoming attuned to his movements and rhythms and patterns; I wonder if anyone else will be able to please me like this. Oh, he is a true artist! He waited what felt like an hour for my first orgasm, and when it happened he kept it going on and on, and with his tongue seemed to control the energy inward and upward. It was as though the climax went inside of me, first deeper inside of my yoni, then deeper inside of my body and upward.

When he does this to me, I make no sound, I do not even breathe. All I can do is feel this heavenly sensation of orgasm going in directions that I cannot logically justify (nor do I try anymore) and the beating of my heart. I hear nothing and feel nothing but the orgasm and my heartbeat, like being back in the womb and his tongue is the umbilical cord to my life.

There will be out there many eager and willing people whom you can practice tantra with. But you will know your true tantric lover. The energy between you will be unlike any other. You may feel a vague remembrance, as though you knew this soul before. His eyes or touch may ring with deep familiarity. Your tantra together will feel better than anything you have ever experienced. It will keep getting better. It will make you feel special, safe, and loved at all times.

Because it involves sex, be wary of people who are involved in tantra with hidden agendas, especially men wanting easy sex. It's a simple matter to learn the buzzwords of tantra and throw around these concepts just to try to impress others. Men like this become particularly tempting when they also happen to be our picture of what we think a lover should be. We must look below the surface and listen beyond their words. Listen to what they say about others, especially about previous partners. How do they hold their lovers, friends, and family in their hearts? There is a wise saying that a man who loves his mother will treat a woman well. (The same is true of a woman who loves her father.) We must carefully analyze our potential tantric partners, using our hearts and our heads.

The main thing to remember is this: A tantric partner should always have our best interest at heart. He will have no agenda or intention other than what is good for you—ever.

The other component is the person's credentials. How long has he been practicing tantra? Has he really been trained to be a teacher of tantra? What is his track record? Just because someone has been practicing tantra for three or five years and has attended a dozen tantra workshops does not mean he or she is even remotely qualified to teach it. We must beware of the people who confidently say, "I can teach you tantra—I've studied it for years!"

My partner went through an extensive training course headed by a tantric teacher by the name of Sunyata Saraswati who had studied in India and co-taught with Bodhi Avinasha. My partner and his wife underwent a tremendous amount of study for many years not just in the discipline of tantra, but in many other modalities as well. Their teaching has tremendous substance. They know what they're talking about. They also walk their talk—that was another indicator that I could rely on and trust them.

In other words, my heart knew from the moment I met my partner that we should be together. But I also used my head to make sure everything was aboveboard.

Ironically, my tantric partner was not at all the picture of my ideal man. I was not physically attracted to him. He was nearly twice my age, overweight, and short. To be perfectly honest, for the two years I waited before starting tantra, I spent much time and energy worrying that he was not what I thought he should be like.

No handsome knight swept me off my feet. Our relationship started in a way utterly different from every other physical relationship with a man that I had ever had. This was not necessarily a bad thing, for I did not have a good history of attracting nice guys. I figured that if they aroused my desire they were good for me. The problem was that my desire was usually aroused by men who were not good for me. I had spent my life going through relationship after relationship, wondering why every guy I met was a jerk. I was always seeking passion. Physical attraction, to me, was love. Emotional closeness was there sometimes, but not always. If I had these two things, I would consider myself fortunate.

What I lacked in my relationships was the spiritual element. When I did meet men who had the same spiritual beliefs, values, and long-term goals, and who saw my potential, and wanted me to fulfill the highest purpose of my soul, I would feel zero chemistry.

Wise friends might say, "But he's the perfect guy!"

My reply would be, "I'm just not physically attracted to him."

Well, of course not. I had not integrated my own physical and emotional self with my spiritual values. How could I possibly find on the outside something I did not have within me?

Stranger still was the form of my tantric relationship. My partner was a tantric teacher, but he was married. A married man! And why would his wife accept this kind of thing?

But love did not remain within the narrow frame of my physical sight or childhood fantasy. I had to expand my vision to encompass the vastness of love. I had to go beyond my perception of what I thought a person should look and be like whom I allowed myself to love.

I got to know his wife very well. Herself a tantric teacher, she was perfectly fine with her husband being my partner. And believe me, I tested her many times to make sure. But this is their life. Tantra is their path, and this is the way they choose to do things. Not all tantric teachers practice with their students. Most teachers who do so will practice with just a few students, and in this case every measure of ensuring safe sex must be strictly maintained.

And so yes, I did think it strange to intensely love and open myself to a friend whom I trusted completely but was not in love with, and on top of that was married.

But of course I could not learn tantra alone. I had considered learning with boyfriends, but whenever I brought up the subject it was obvious they just liked the idea that it involved sex. I could have told them I wanted us to howl at the Moon every night and they would have said, "Great!"—as long as it involved sex.

I wanted to learn tantra so much that I decided to let go of all my pre-conceived notions and take a leap of faith.

My partner is one of the most giving men I have ever met. I get the feel-ing that he is constantly thinking, "How can I make her happier?" He has taught me more about love than anyone else, not from his words but by his actions. He gives of his heart more than I had ever experienced before. He gives by listening to my problems, both petty and serious. No matter how busy he is, he will always have time if I need him. He has become my best friend. He rarely says no to anything I ask of him.

He puts up with all of my idiosyncrasies, all of the times I've pushed him away because I feared intimacy. I sometimes wonder how someone could love me so unconditionally, with all the flaws I have. I can be demanding, self-absorbed, moody, and aloof. But he is always there. He doesn't try to change me, for he loves me exactly as I am, and if I never evolved or changed one bit for the rest of my life, he would still love me unconditionally. At the same time, he sees my potential, beyond even what I can see. He sees the seeds of talent within me and patiently reminds me, again and again, that is who I am. He has helped me become greater than I ever thought I could be. There is no one in this world who knows me better than my partner. He is a soul mate.

Thus, with this amount of trust and safety, I could practice tantra with him because I knew he would never, ever hurt me. I knew he would never, ever leave me. I knew he would always be there for me.

Soon I realized that the relationship's lack of romance made me feel safe—because of my own fears of intimacy. Although he was emotionally and spiri-tually and physically there for me, my partner was married. I didn't have to commit my life to this person. It turns out that I had a huge, immense fear of commitment. This relationship let me work on other areas of myself without requiring that I confront that issue up front.

With a focused intention of love, ours was a spiritual bond right from the start. During tantra I could easily concentrate upon my spiritual purpose without getting lost in the passion of the moment. I discovered shortly that I had big issues about uniting my spiritual life with my sexual life. Tantra, being all about merging these aspects, would of course push every button I had. But in the beginning it felt safer to start from a context that appeared to separate the two.

The normal expectations that, in a normal relationship, can tie us down like prisoners did not exist between us. Each time we were together, we had a clean canvas on which to paint.

Through this relationship I could safely open up and expose all my fear and resistance. There was nothing to prove. There were no games to play or agendas to fulfill. I knew I was safe enough to take an honest look at my real feelings about sex and my sexuality, and at how I felt about myself as a woman. And there were a lot of fears that I was to uncover. It seems I didn't know myself as well as I'd thought.

Love knew what it was doing, after all.

I continued for years practicing tantra with this man without thinking of him as a boyfriend or life partner. I had several committed relationships concurrent with our tantric practice. This was challenging for me: most men did not understand why I chose to live this way. Some would leave. Some would grudgingly tolerate it. It's one thing to commit to a religion and go to church every Sunday. It's quite another to spend that Sunday practicing tantra with another person. I felt alone in my choice, especially because I couldn't really talk about it.

I can see now that I was attracting relationships that did not support my tantric path because parts of me felt torn about being tantric. For years I was ambivalent about my lifestyle, keeping one foot in each world: one foot in my "reality" of family, friends, and work, and one foot in my "spirituality," which felt like the very purpose for my existence. I felt guilty about dividing these two parts of myself, as though I was hiding something from friends and family. I felt like an outsider.

I know of tantrics who live within a supportive tantric community. But

I didn't want to hide out in a sequestered group. I'm a city girl (or at least suburban). I'm active in my worldly activities. I have ambitions for a career and financial independence. I want to be an integral part of my family. I am not just tantric.

I wanted to belong in this world. Yet I also knew that tantra is for me. I knew it to the marrow.

One day I came across one of the final chapters of *Tantra: The Cult of the Feminine* by Andre Van Lysebeth. Here I discovered the words that explained the very relationship between my partner and me:

> Meeting the guru is an unpredictable event, but when it occurs, it changes life for both, and is as indelible as a tattoo: one can divorce one's wife, never one's guru. The *guru-chela relationship* involving a man and a woman often implies actual sexual practices whose intensity goes far beyond what is ordinarily experienced. Most of the time, however, they do not live together—they can lead a distinct sex life with their "normal" partner without becoming jealous. The guru-chela relationship, far from destroying the relationship of a settled couple, can on the contrary make it stronger and more lasting. Whatever is characteristic of a normal love relationship (possessiveness, jealousy, etc.) does not exist in theirs, and their bond is similar to that which exists between twins. This is probably what makes theirs a stable, lasting relationship. Their relationship transcends time and space: mysteriously, they are always in contact with each other on a subtle, spiritual plane, just as twins are. During their daily meditation, they contact each other, sometimes even without being conscious of it. Their beings remain linked forever, maybe even beyond death.*

From simply a physical perspective, the tantra we practiced was absolutely amazing. Even though we lacked emotional passion, the levels of energy that we created in bed were incredible. We have a chemistry together that I had never felt before.

But even beyond the sexual aspect, we share a deep connection. We feel

---

*Andre Van Lysebeth, *Tantra: The Cult of the Feminine* (York Beach, Maine: Samuel Weiser, 1995): 344–45.

the energy between us now even when we're not engaged in tantra. When we're sitting on opposite ends of a couch, fully clothed, discussing mundane details of the day, there's electricity between us. It is a thick, pervasive warmth. It causes us both to start sweating. It is a sweetness, a tenderness, an endless trust. We know each other's hearts.

How did we arrive at such closeness? Not easily. It took me years to become comfortable with just our physical relationship. But doing tantra for only physical pleasure is like having a huge feast in front of you and merely tasting a morsel of leftover bread. And one day I could no longer delay my lesson. It was time for me to merge my sexuality with my spirituality, and I knew it. Flashes of passion began to rise to the surface of our relationship.

But my fear of love overwhelmed me, and I tried to ignore these emerging emotions. Why would I want to push away any feelings of romance, the same feelings that I so desperately sought in my usual relationships with men?

At first I thought it was because he was, after all, married. One day I went to his wife, feeling quite upset and guilty, and I told her my predicament. I said I was starting to feel things I didn't want to feel, or thought I shouldn't feel.

She looked into my eyes and softly said, "Why do you think I would not want you to feel passion for my husband? He is your tantric teacher. The path of tantra is about passion, my dear."

But even with her blessing I still argued with myself, insisting that I wanted to retain the purity of our spiritual tantric relationship. Taken alone, I could understand sexuality. Or love. Or my relationship with God. But combining these parts of me? I was confused. It did not compute. And there were good reasons, I would soon discover, that it did not compute for me. I had to change nearly the entire context from which I perceived my life. I finally had to face the terror of combining the three elements of spirituality, sexuality, and passionate love.

Part 2

Mastering the Self

Surrender and Creation
7

*M*y perceptions are becoming fluid. I am dissociating myself from the collection of thoughts, emotions, and experiences that make me who I am. But who I am is so vastly different from what I thought! Like the phoenix rising from the ashes, so my soul rises from my binding and temporal thoughts. And through this I am learning. And every step is a joy!

"With your permission, I will turn your body into one big clit."

These are the words whispered by my tantric partner shortly after my initiation. He was only partly joking.

Tantra embraces the opposing actions of will and passivity. Paradoxically, we are expanding outward, becoming more of love and God, while at the same time releasing everything within us that causes pain and suffering. It is a building up of all that is and a surrender of all that is not.

This is a path not of pleasure but of extreme pleasure.

Few methods of self-transformation or spirituality begin from a place of positivity. Psychotherapy, for example, heals by focusing on our past traumas. Catholicism tends to highlight our inherent sinfulness. Psychotherapy, Catholicism, and tantra can easily have the same positive purpose of healing and personal betterment. But tantra begins with the positive and uses the positive throughout.

Tantra embraces the concept that God feels good. In Eastern spirituality enlightened beings, such as the laughing Buddha, are often portrayed as being incredibly happy. Spiritual moments can eradicate physical pain. Many people have recalled near-death experiences as feeling close to God with an overwhelming sense of euphoria.* Years ago a group of children testify to have sighted the Virgin Mary in Fatima. The children would be in such a trance during these visions that they wouldn't feel pins stuck into them.

But not all of us equate a life devoted to God with happiness and ecstasy. Western religious art depicts many weeping martyrs and saints being stoned to death or led to execution. I learned that God could be merciful if you prayed a lot. But He could also be a wrathful avenger. I was taught that God was outside me, and thus I was skeptical that all experience of God is pure bliss. The method of tantra, as we know, uses sexual pleasure to increase pleasure in all aspects of consciousness, both body and spirit. When the mind is properly focused, physical pleasure will increase emotional satisfaction and spiritual fulfillment.

Sexual pleasure increases and then is channeled to expose and burn away the pain within us. As negativity diminishes, it is replaced by cellular memories of pleasure. Over time, the body will consistently feel more pleasure than pain—vastly, vastly more pleasure. Thus, the tool we use to heal the pain is sexual pleasure through the physical body, but doing so affects all aspects of the psyche. The pain I'm referring to healing herein can be emotional as well as physical—feelings of lack, desperation, sadness, hurt.

Increasing Pleasure

Experts have determined that we use less than 10 percent of the brain. It may follow that we experience an equally nominal amount of our capacity for sexual pleasure. Only recently has research revealed that the nerve structure of the female sex organ is completely unlike that which the revered

---

*This phenomenon is not just emotional, but can be physiological as well; upon dying, the brain actually generates hormones that produce an effect of ecstasy or euphoria.

medical reference *Gray's Anatomy* has described for years.* In fact, the size of the clitoris is "at least twice as large as most anatomy texts show, and tens of times larger than the average person realizes."† How little we know about ourselves, especially our sexuality!

The first step of tantra is to increase our physical capacity for pleasure. We train the body to give and receive pleasure in higher and higher volumes. For example, our physical vision is able to see a range of electromagnetic waves called the color spectrum. The color spectrum is only a tiny portion of the electromagnetic spectrum. What if our eyes could see beyond the small portion of this spectrum that we now know? What if there were more colors out there that, if trained, our eyes could see? Tantra expands our spectrum of what we know as pleasure—the pleasure spectrum, if you will. There are infinite ways to experience physical pleasure, and each experience is a life unto itself.

Expanding the Radius

The region where we feel sensations of sexual pleasure will slowly spread out from just the clitoris or penis, so that the surrounding areas become just as sensitized as the sexual organ. The inner thighs and perineum become as sensitive as the actual sex organ, so one can actually have an orgasm in areas of the body other than the genitals. The inner thighs can reach orgasm. The anus can reach orgasm. The outer labia can reach orgasm. Every part of the body can be trained to reach orgasm.

The orgasm of each area will feel different, and certain areas of the body will achieve more intense orgasms. The entire body can be trained to be orgasmic, because orgasms physically occur in the brain. It's true: The brain is the biggest sex organ in the body. We want to get to the point where the slightest pressure, touch, or thought can trigger an orgasm. In fact, there have been documented medical cases in which only the physiological activity of

*Henry Gray, *Gray's Anatomy: The Anatomical Basis of Medicine and Surgery* (Kent, UK: Churchill Livingstone, 1995).
†"Durex Global Sex Survey" (Cheshire, UK: SSL International, 1997).

the brain can trigger an orgasm.*

I'll never forget the first time my partner made my inner thigh, about one inch below the point where the leg begins, achieve orgasm. That one little spot! It was then that I began to realize how many little spots there are just waiting to come alive.

When our partners can look at us from across the room and give us an orgasm, we are well on our way to increasing our physical capacity for pleasure!

Deepening the Pleasure

As the orgasmic areas of the body spread, the pleasure will likewise deepen within the body. Pleasure will penetrate beneath the topical skin, into its deeper layers, and into the nerves, and into the blood, and into the internal organs, and into the deepest marrow. All the cells of our bodies become part of the orgasmic symphony.

I feel my whole body becoming juiced and lubricated. My heart pounding, my blood pulsing, the nerves everywhere in my body sensitizing, the pleasure working its way deep inside me. It is a vital essence, the energy of youth, renewing every part of my body, as though I could live three hundred years more!

Lengthening the Time

The worldwide average duration for sex is less than eighteen minutes.† Tantra intensifies pleasure by slowly increasing the energies of pleasure within the body. It is because of this slow process, necessary to build energy, that the average tantric session needs to last from one to three hours. My longest tantric experience was seven hours nonstop!

---

*In "Why Women's Orgasms Are on a Higher Plane," Jeremy Laurence describes medical examples in which an epileptic seizure causes the experience of orgasm, especially so in women (*Independent,* 12 December 1997, p. 2).

†Susan Williamson, "The Truth About Women," *New Scientist,* August 1998, vol. 159, no. 2145.

Building the Orgasm

But practicing tantra for many hours will not bring results unless we skillfully learn how to build up the orgasm. *Building the orgasm is one of the most important techniques in tantra.* The man gets his partner as close to orgasm as possible and keeps her on that plateau, not allowing an orgasm, by changing rhythm, slowing the pace, or decreasing pressure. Once she cools off to the point where he knows she won't go over that edge, the partners repeat the process. He builds her orgasm, gets her as close as possible without going over the edge, and maintains her on that plateau just before orgasm. We want to do this a minimum of three times, but this practice can easily continue for an hour. Each time partners build, they are bringing each other higher.

The technique of building the orgasm does not mean having foreplay for a long time. There is a world of difference between merely exciting our partner and learning how to build up the orgasm. For example, if a man is performing oral sex on me for a solid hour and is not building up the orgasm, I might reach a level of arousal but then plateau. If I remain at the same level of arousal for too long without getting more excited, my body will go on automatic pilot —the body gets bored, in a way. The key is *building*. There should always be an upward progression to the level of excitement.

The secret to building the orgasm is knowing precisely when our partners intend to orgasm. The closer we can bring them to orgasm, without taking them over that edge of ecstasy, the stronger we will build the orgasm. When we can thus master their rhythms, we will be able to launch our partners into orbit!

Mastering the first build is the most critical part. Once we do that, it will be relatively easy to continue to build the orgasm for as long as we want. This all happens within the first fifteen minutes or so of foreplay. My goal is to get my partner to forget about everything in this world except me (and my tongue). Sometimes my partner's body responds to everything I do, and he is so ready for tantra that he would practically achieve orgasm if I breathed on his nipple! But sometimes his mind is on other things and he is somewhat distracted by the day, or he ate too much and his blood is busy helping him digest.

Whatever the situation, the key is the first build. I begin to lick his lingam. If he's really responsive, I know it instantly because of how hard he gets. If he's unfocused, he might need a little more pressure and stimulation so that he becomes more intent. I want to be at the point, within the first five to fifteen minutes, at which I know without a doubt that I can make him achieve orgasm at any moment. If he is really excited, then I know I already have the ability to do this. If I am not absolutely sure that I can make him climax, I need to get there. This might take me more time, and it might take some adjustment of my technique. But I keep working at it until I know he is ready. Once I'm there, everything is smooth sailing. I want to use the *least amount of pressure needed* to keep him excited; too much pressure desensitizes the genitals. (Men keep thinking that they must act like a living vibrator by pounding away as fast and as hard as they can! In some ways, a woman's worst enemy is the vibrator, because it desensitizes the vaginal canal. Of course, some women would never have any enjoyment without the skill of that device, and this is a very unfortunate predicament to be in!)

When I first began tantra, my yoni was very desensitized. The first time my partner gave me oral sex, he needed to press on my yoni rather hard, because I couldn't feel it any other way. It must have taken more than an hour just for me to relax enough to have an orgasm. He had not mastered my rhythms because I was not letting him do so. But soon thereafter, my partner was able to use less and less pressure, to the point where he didn't even need to touch my clitoris for me to have an orgasm. My yoni has basically been made anew. It has become extremely sensitive and extremely responsive. And it feels so much better this way!

When first beginning tantra with a new partner, we will most likely need to use a lot of pressure if that is what he or she is accustomed to. But over time we will be able to make our partners more aroused with less stimulation.

Some keys to remember about pressure are as follows. If we speed up the movement of our tongues, we must use less pressure, and if we decrease the speed, we use more pressure (not a lot of pressure, just a little more). Also, once a woman has an orgasm, it is essential to back off, by using less pressure and going very slowly. This allows the area that has climaxed to reintegrate.

After a clitoral orgasm, in particular, the clitoris is too sensitive to have any pressure on it. Thus it is good to move the tongue to other areas of the yoni, such as the inner and outer lips. After four or five orgasms on the outside of the yoni, go back to the clitoris for a finale. When at last there is a second clitoral orgasm after all of this buildup, the orgasm just goes on and on.

Here is a summary of the steps to building the orgasm:

1. Building the orgasm occurs during foreplay, such as oral pleasuring.
2. The first build—the most important—requires that we stimulate our partners until we know they are just about to achieve orgasm.
3. Just before orgasm, we change rhythm, pressure, or tempo so that our partners do not reach orgasm but instead linger at that pre-orgasm plateau for a couple of minutes.
4. When we know they will not have an orgasm, we again begin the progressive building upward and repeat the process.
5. Building the orgasm requires that our partners become progressively more excited (and not plateau).
6. We should use the least amount of pressure required to continue the increased arousal.
7. We repeat this process a minimum of three times.
8. Each time we reach the pre-orgasm stage, we will be raising our partners' orgasm level higher and higher.

This technique is a means to becoming one with the patterns of our partners— and the result is sensationally huge orgasms.

Multiple Orgasms

As if sensationally huge orgasms are not enough, we can also increase the number of orgasms that our partners have. Women can have an unlimited number. There are many ways in which a woman's body can achieve orgasm. Vast varieties of level, texture, and hue can color the landscape of our temples. (But you need to wait for chapter 9 for the details—see, I'm building the energy for you).

It has gotten to the point where my orgasms are so large that, deep into hours of lovemaking, I do not know any longer whether or not my body is orgasming, as I am in such a constantly aroused state. My cells tingle. My muscles pulse in orgasmic rhythm. But then, just when I think it can't get any better, my partner will really amaze me by giving me an even bigger orgasm.

Because men can achieve orgasm only once or twice on average, we compensate by doing the aforementioned, the building of the orgasm and keeping him at the plateau and then building upward again. When we are doing this correctly, at some point the man will begin to secrete a steady stream of clear fluid,* which continues the entire time of stimulation.

In Taoism it is thought that when a man has an orgasm, he is actually losing the vital essence that will keep him youthful and healthy. Some tantrics believe that it is not necessary for a grown man to orgasm at all, or that he should limit himself to once every couple of weeks. In this case we will focus only on building the orgasm. Apparently this practice of not climaxing makes some men feel energized. My teacher and his wife teach that a man can achieve the same amount of heightened energy providing his partner can do the buildup skillfully. It also depends on the age of the man and his level of libido. Younger men, for example, may have a lot more sexual energy.

In our practice, I almost always bring my partner all the way to orgasm after a long buildup. As he achieves orgasm, he pulls energy into his body and upward, so while he is secreting his semen, mentally and energetically he is pulling energy inward, filling his body with vitality. This seems to effectively energize him.

Increasing the Duration

We can also increase the length of time that the physical orgasm occurs. An average orgasm might last ten seconds. In tantra we want to draw this out to minutes, then to tens of minutes, and then to an hour. Again, the key is in the buildup. It is crucial to sensitize the genitals and the surrounding areas. The buildup will naturally cause a larger, longer orgasm. During the orgasm we can also keep it going by being one with our partners' rhythms. Every orgasm has a rhythm. We can match the rhythm through pace and pressure, and keep it going by continuing that heightened rhythm.

---

*This is the transparent, pre-seminal fluid that flows prior to ejaculation.

The Beginning of Oneness

Increasing, expanding, deepening, building: through all actions of tantra we seek to produce oneness. In the beginning we seek physical oneness—to know our partners' bodies as if they were our own. At first all we strive for are moments of oneness with our partners. Then we work on extending these moments so that each tantric union becomes several hours of blissful, heavenly oneness.

Physical oneness leads to emotional oneness. When combined with emotion, physical pleasure transforms into passion. Passion is the fire of life and the fire of a relationship. Passion is romantic love, but it's much more. It is the substance within us that motivates our compassion for others, our concern for humanity, our determination to maintain positive relationships year after year, in spite of all life's turmoil. Passion is the language of the heart.

Once emotional oneness is established, we strive for spiritual oneness. We channel our physical and emotional passion inward: into the hearts and souls of our partners, and into the hearts and souls of ourselves. We use passion to fuel our purpose, which as we know by now is to transcend our limited awareness and embody God more deeply.

To the untrained eye, tantra can seem somewhat slow, almost uneventful. Contrary to what many people think, tantra is not about mastering a multitude of sexual positions, as illustrated in texts such as the *Kama-sutra*.

My partner might be performing oral sex on me for two hours, his tongue slowly moving with utmost delicacy over every little detail of my yoni. He will take a small area of my yoni—for instance, a tiny fold on the right inner labium—and softly tease it with his tongue for twenty minutes, until this little spot is swollen to three times its normal size. This small part of my yoni could have an orgasm at any moment. Then he switches to another little spot. Perhaps now it is a tiny fold on the left side of my inner labia. As he is performing cunnilingus on me, as I am silently lying there, deeply breathing, much is going on within my body and my mind. In my body I am bringing up the energy into my higher chakras. With my mind I am opening my heart to my partner, to the incredible amount of love he has for me.

Tantra is distinctly different from normal lovemaking because of the concentration on the breath and the channeling of energy. Directing energy accomplishes two things. First, it requires great focus to be totally present. Second, it gives purpose and direction to our practice.

As we practice tantra, we visualize the movement of energy in the mind's eye. There are a number of ways to visualize the circuit of energy. We might visualize this energy coming into our bodies through the root chakra. It then travels upward along the inside of the spine, through each chakra, into the heart, and then outward into our partners. We send it into our partners through our hands, through our tongues, through our hearts. When we bring it up from the genitals and into the higher places of the body, we will feel grounded. We can also pull energy from the crown chakra (top of the head), down through the body and out our genitals and into our partners' genitals. Pulling energy from the heavens feels completely different; it makes us feel vast and airy.

Some see energy as an aspect of God, or pure consciousness, or the creative force of the universe. It can reflect the aspects of the self—that is, the energy being pulled up from the earth is feminine, and the energy pulled down from the heavens is masculine. The energy might be a bright color or it might be pure white light. We visualize our bodies becoming one, seeing not two separate bodies giving and receiving energy but instead one body that is working as a single unit. When the energy of two people combines into one, it takes on its own life. It creates a sensation very different from what arises when either person is using energy alone. There have been times during lovemaking when I physically cannot feel where my skin ends and my partner's begins.

We combine our visualization of energy with breathing. As we inhale, we pull the energy upward into our bodies. As we exhale, we send the energy out into our partners. Both partners breathe in unison. We can rotate the inhalation and exhalation, such that when one person is inhaling, the other is simultaneously exhaling. When we breathe through the nose, we focus our minds. When we breathe through the mouth, we become more grounded in our bodies.

Kundalini responds to the current of energy and breathing that we generate again and again through tantra. One day—after weeks or years—our kundalini will awaken. If we have properly prepared our minds and bodies for its activation, through other disciplines and with the instruction of a good teacher, kundalini will be a wonderful complement to our practice of tantra. Kundalini greatly increases the pleasure we feel because it gives us even more energy to draw from. Ideally, both partners will have awakened kundalini. Once that happens, look out, because pleasure will pour forth in torrents and transformation will accelerate.

The pleasure, now taking the form of kundalini, will rise up through each of our chakras. Every time another chakra comes into the orgasm, the sweeter the physical pleasure, the deeper the spiritual pleasure, the more the heart will open and the emotions will lift. Tantra is an ascending path of happiness, so our highs become higher, and our lows are less low.

Love is about giving of ourselves. During tantra we have a single-minded goal to give our partners as much pleasure as possible. We give through use of pressure, rhythm, and pace. When we are sexually pleasuring our partners, and concentrating on nothing but desire in this moment, an amazing thing happens. We learn how to love more deeply. We learn how pleasurable it is to love unconditionally.

Tantra is a singular meditation of two people. The focus really becomes the unspoken connection and communication between partners. Our thoughts become one. In this state we experience deep empathy, for we cannot hate another whom we are at one with.

The sole object of tantric meditation (see chapter 8) is our partners' happiness. The sole purpose of tantric meditation is to discover how to develop that happiness into extreme joy a thousand times over. Our partners' happiness is our only concern.

Surrendering Fear

As we use tantra to increase the many facets of pleasure within our bodies, emotions, and spirit, an interesting phenomenon happens. Tantra pushes up to the surface everything that resists pleasure.

Any path, I logically reasoned, that uses sexual pleasure to bring me to enlightenment must be easy!

Simple, yes. Easy? Not exactly.

To my great astonishment, only months into my tantric practice I found myself staring at a woman in the mirror who had more fear of pleasure than I thought humanly possible.

The truth is, I had lots of nasty thoughts about sex. In fact, I don't think any negative association with sex escaped my permeable mind. But there they were, the naked and unedited truths about what I felt about sex. In my mind, sex did not equate to love. Sex could mean many things. Sex, in its worst form, could mean possession, abuse, even rape. Pleasure could be pain. Love could be hate.

Part of my subconscious had defined sex as a purely physical experience that could be devoid of love, and in fact might be more pleasurable if there was no love involved. Perhaps it is the primitive part of us that can seek animalistic sex over love. Combined with the general social attitude that sex is dirty and bad—remnants of childhood—this left my impressionable self little room for hope.

The nurturing nature of tantric lovemaking was a contradiction to me. It was one thing to read about sex, and to think about it at night when alone, and to fantasize about it until my body felt warmed. But it was quite another to practice tantra in the light of day, with another person who is sending currents of energy and love into my body. I loved tantra; who wouldn't love something that is so fully pleasurable? But at the same time I feared it more than anything else.

How could I both love and fear at the same time? How could I simultaneously hold opposing thoughts in my mind and yet feel perfectly normal about it? How did I get to this point where sex and love were a contradiction in my mind? Was it society's twisted views about sex? Did my religious upbringing mess me up that badly? Were these thoughts inherited from my family?

Nevertheless, here I was. How I had acquired these feelings did not really matter now. My biggest concern was how I would overcome them.

My fear never seemed to come up while we were practicing tantra; it always materialized before we started. One day I was lying in bed with my partner. I didn't want to practice tantra. I felt shy about his touch. I couldn't look into his eyes. He sensed my trepidation and asked me what was wrong.

Did I dare open up to him? Did I dare reveal my darkest feelings about sex?

Teary-eyed, I decided to confide in my partner, as we lay there in bed, about all my self-loathing and dread of sex. I told him things I had never told anyone else before.

He didn't flinch. He didn't throw me out of the room in disgust. He simply said, "Well, that's common. Are you doing tantric meditation as we practice tantra?"

Uh, no.

Instead of meditating I had been distancing myself from my partner by evoking fantasies. I would fantasize about any sexual experience—the kinkier the better. I thought I did this because I was such a visual and sexual person. In truth it was escapism. It protected me from intimacy. It allowed me to be sexually open without getting any emotions involved.

All along, my thoughts about sex being wrong and bad were covering up the real issue that lurked underneath. The real issue was my fear of love and oneness.

Intention is key, as my partner pointed out. If we practice tantra without intention, we allow the energy to release in lots of directions. Without intention we are not controlling our own transformation. If I have nonloving thoughts about myself, tantra will not force me to change. Tantra simply shows me what is already in my mind. Tantric meditation grounds the intention of love, making it more than just a concept in a book.

Of course, then I felt guilty that I was not practicing tantric meditation as I should be. And so I shared my immense guilt.

"You're very hard on yourself," he said.

Seeing his confidence in me, I took a deep breath and, with my mind and heart, made an internal commitment to stop beating myself up and just let it be okay.

Besides, it's very difficult to stay fearful and guilty while having an hour-long orgasm.

Tantric
Meditation

looked within my heart to see what I would find. I glimpsed my Center—a tiny, tiny dot, a white hole extending infinitely deep. I stopped, because I could go no farther. I had not earned that right. I respected her boundaries and encircled my energy around this jewel at the center of my being. It welcomed my embrace, was glad to have the attention.

During the first months of tantra, it is important simply to develop discipline: employ whatever means are necessary to practice tantra consistently. So although I started practicing tantra without any kind of tantric meditation, this was necessary for me just to establish habit. That way, I could first get accustomed to the rituals, learn my patterns and those of my partner, and acclimatize my body and mind to immense energy levels.

Tantra stirred up many feelings. The first step was to acknowledge these feelings without suppression. But that took me only so far. If the mind is going to let go of a negative feeling, there must be something else to replace that feeling, or else there is a tendency to go back to the way things were. I had to do two things: surrender my negative thoughts and then fill the void with something positive. I had to create other associations.

Tantric meditation would be the tool to create my feelings anew. It took me to the next level, helping me to unlearn some bad emotional habits I had acquired over the past fifteen-plus years. One particularly detrimental habit was a tendency to remain emotionally separate from others. Through tantric meditation, I would learn how to link my sexuality with my heart and take this loving passion into my relationship with God.

I resisted tantric meditation. I wanted only to drown in physical ecstasy. Tantric lovemaking can be very distracting because it feels so good. It took years to develop consistency in my meditations.

Tantric meditation is the means of attaining tantra's final requisite: a consistent intention of love. In tantric meditation we listen to God. We open our minds. We tap into the collective creative source, going beyond our limiting thoughts, and hear God. God's sweet symphony can always be heard, but we must open our untrained ears to the right chords.

In tantric meditation we concentrate on the physical, the emotional, and the spiritual simultaneously. Our focus is both active and passive. Each part of the tantric act is predisposed toward certain meditation techniques. There are some books that describe tantric meditation in great detail, but most of the meditations I use came to me without any instruction. My tantric teacher did not sit me down and say, "Do this, do that," while we practiced tantra. I learned the basics about breathing, ritual, energy flow, and intention beforehand, and then we got together and practiced. Ours was more of a silent teaching while we practiced tantra. And isn't that the way it should be? Who wants to practice tantric lovemaking while getting a bunch of instructions!

Constant words of instruction were not necessary between us also because my partner did not need to teach me his technique. He was not trying to make me into a great male tantric who could raise a woman's energy levels. He was doing techniques that helped me to embody my own enlightenment so I would become a receptive female tantrika. There were many times when, after we were finished, I would ask, "How on earth did you do that?"

He would jokingly respond, "Well, if I tell you I'll give away my secrets." The truth is, I didn't need to understand his technique, because if I were to spend all my time wondering how he was doing things, I would have the tendency to analyze the tantra rather than simply be in the moment and enjoy the process. There are experiences of tantra that don't need to be put into words.

Generally, the flow of a single tantric meditation will go as follows:

1. Physical: total concentration on the physical pleasure in the moment
2. Emotional: immersion in loving thoughts and worship of our partner's divinity
3. Spiritual: feeling ourselves and our partner as a single unit that is connected to spirit, or God

Physical Awakening

After we have shared our ritual preparation, my partner and I slip into bed and hold each other, breathing together. We gently kiss and caress each other's bodies. My partner kisses my lips, neck, arms, nipples, stomach, and thighs, sometimes my feet, backs of my knees, calves, back, buttocks, shoulders.

My partner is a master of energy control. As he pleasures me with oral stimulation, he is bringing up energy from his root chakra along his spine, out from his heart, through his tongue and hands. I feel an electricity coming out of him and into me.

I meditate on the sexual energy within my body and between us. In my mind I'm feeling, seeing, and sensing only the experience of this sexual foreplay. I concentrate on his tongue and the skin directly underneath, each stroke feeling uniquely magnificent to the skin being caressed. I delve into the details of my skin—how each inch, fold, and cell engorges with pleasure. I feel the shape and texture of his tongue, the pressure as it moves, the rate at which it slowly and steadily explores me. A thin layer of soft moisture lies between my skin and his tongue. My yoni feels the beating of his heart pounding through his tongue. Each portion of my yoni's delicate skin begins to swell and expand, opening and warming.

Up inside my yoni, my walls are moistening and enlarging, and my cherished G spot is beginning to grow. I can almost hear it calling for attention, asking for touch, reaching outward, seeking pleasure. My partner licks me from my knees, up my inner thighs, onto every piece of my yoni, not neglecting a spot. Each area that he pleasures swells, and with this size grows an intoxicating ecstasy. I now visualize my yoni and his tongue growing very large. My outer labia swell, my inner lips open, my clitoris turns a hard, ruby red. Now in my mind I expand my yoni and his tongue, so that I begin to meditate on more and more specific details of both of us. The more details I see, the more places into which that pleasure sinks its way.

I visualize my sexuality as three times its natural size, in vivid detail. The individual nerves on my skin pulsate in ecstasy. With every touch of his tongue the cells of my yoni expand and engorge.

When my partner brings me to first climax, after perhaps an hour, orgasmic waves overwhelm my body. Each area of my yoni—the lips, the inner walls, my clit—is having its own unique rhythmic rippling of pleasure, a subset that is convulsing in perfect harmony with the waves of orgasm surging through my whole body, from head to toe.

Emotional Connection

Dwelling in this euphoric flow, my partner begins anew to build up the pleasure within me, starting this time from the higher place where I am now. As he increases this energy, I channel the sexual energy and my consciousness into my heart, linking one chakra to the other—the pleasure to the love—so that both become one, both are contained within the other. As my heart begins to warm and grow with ecstatic pleasure, I sink deeper into it, deep inside. In my heart I see a very small core, only the size of a marble yet as bright as the sun. I take my mind into this core and am overwhelmed by its softness, its warmth, its vulnerability and openness. This is the part of me that I have shielded with layer upon layer of armor, the part I have so often feared. It is my core, my essence. It is I, shining in a brilliance that I remember only faintly. It's hard to stay in this place within my heart—I feel as though I will burst with joy—so I let the vast amount of sexual energy assist me. I focus here, letting my consciousness get used to being close to me.

I now see the light of my heart's core growing larger, brighter, its rays reaching out farther, to the surface of my body and through my skin. I am radiating with my own essence and the pleasure continues to increase until my partner blesses my body with a second orgasm. This time my orgasm is deeper, now both physical and heartfelt, emotional, connecting me to my essence, increasing my heart's capacity—each wave of orgasm sends pleasure into my heart, cleansing it, washing it clean with the pure energy of God.

Many orgasms later I will reverse the energy flow so that I can give back all that my partner has given me and more. He lies next to me, we kiss intimately, and my body explores his. I give my softness to him, I give my energy to him, through my touch, my kiss, my body. I bring my mouth down to his lingam, the place from which I will worship him for what will feel both an eternity and a timeless moment.

I turn my entire perception, mind, and senses on my partner. I gently touch his awakened manhood, stroking his lingam and his scrotum, his soft perineum, the opening of his anus. I let my sight open up to him, my listening, my sense of smell, my touch. Now I taste him. I begin very slowly, one hand gently massaging his testes upward while my tongue is on his shaft. I begin at the base of his erect lingam and slowly move upward, feeling his smooth firmness with my tongue. Each area of his lingam is different—some parts are smooth and some are rough. Each ridge I explore, each small area of skin—I listen to each part for what it wants. Each part asks for something different: sometimes more pressure, sometimes a slower rhythm.

I move very slowly. I dance my tongue over to the left side of his lingam. I am feeling veins that grow larger under my stroking tongue. I notice now that the fleshy skin on the anterior of his penis is textured—it responds strongly to me. It is craving a careful touch. It has been anticipating my tongue so much that all I must do is gently lick in a circular pattern and the skin expands underneath my tongue, enlarging as to beckon me to touch more of it. Now my tongue reaches the bottom ridge of the head of the lingam and my partner moans. I listen to what the ridge desires and fulfill it just a bit more slowly than what it wants, for I know this lingam is ready to burst and yet I still wish to build the energy. I now shift to the right side of the shaft, and it seems that the right side has been anticipating me even more. The right side feels unique. Again I listen through my tongue and soon he is breathing quite heavily, again moaning. When my tongue slides onto the bottom portion of his shaft and slowly licks upward just slightly onto the head of his lingam, he moans louder and his scrotum tightens.

I continue this for a while, keeping his excitement at a constant level, making sure his heartbeat remains at this same rate. I must maintain a delicate balance within him, knowing him enough so that I steadily bring him higher and higher, but not in a way that he will go over the edge. I know that he could achieve orgasm at any time if I merely increased the pressure or rate slightly, for I can feel this in his skin and in his breathing, so I must focus even more.

Now that he is thoroughly aroused, I bring my consciousness briefly into my own body. I am buzzing with thick energy from his pleasuring me, and I draw forth this energy from my root chakra, up the center of my spine, through my heart, and send it out my tongue into him. A silver light rises upward from my spine, through my tongue, and into his sexuality, up his spine and directly into the center of his heart. After several repetitions, the silver light takes on a life of its own and automatically lifts from within me and into him, as automatic as breathing.

I again tease the most sensitive part of his penis, the fleshy protrusion on the anterior of his lingam just below the head. As I lay my moist tongue on this precious jewel, I look at his face and see his eyes rolling upward. He is smiling, and I focus my gaze on his heart, visualizing my energy going upward through his lingam into his heart, filling his body with love. I can see his heart chakra! Rising from his chest, it is pure white and opened wide like a flower, a white lotus with a thousand gentle petals. I am concentrating now on both his body filling with energy and the heightened state of his arousal. When he is less than a moment from orgasm, I change the stroking pattern of my tongue. He sighs heavily. I continue to raise him to the point just before orgasm—mere milliseconds—then decrease or change the intensity.

My goal is to bring him as near to orgasm as possible and then stop. Again, I build him up and then stop. Each time I get him almost to the point of orgasm and I then back down; I am raising him to a higher plateau. At each interval his pleasure is growing more and more. He now begins to secrete his sweet juice. It flows into my mouth and tastes like it is charged with electricity. It tickles my tongue. My desire is that he remain at such a peak level that he continues to secrete this nectar for hours on end.

I feel myself becoming wetter and wetter, being pleasured by pleasuring him. I must remain at one with his rhythms. And now it is so easy for me to see into his heart. I can read his thoughts. I feel his pleasure within my own body. I feel a deep love for him. I want his happiness more than life itself.

Spiritual Completion

Both immersed in the energy of us, it is now time to invite God into our passion. My partner asks permission to go inside me, and I accept hungrily and passionately. We begin in perfect stillness. Without any hip movement, using only the muscles within my yoni, I squeeze down upon him with each rung of muscle.* I bring him in, and in so doing I feel his breath deepen and my own pleasure swelling. We set our minds on our sexual place of merging, letting this sensation of pleasure increase. We are on fire! Again we listen to each other, hearing the sexual desire of the other, and respond simultaneously. Our desires blend and somehow merge into one. We move easily, in this single rhythm created from the two of us, the energy now filling into a deep passion.

My G-spot throbs in pleasure, and I climax again and again, my entire body shuddering and convulsing. His eyes are lit with love and fire. We are closing the circuit, a perfect circle of energy going through one and then the other, simultaneously giving and receiving. I'm wondering where his body ends and mine begins, and then I don't care anymore.

We are meditating upon us. We see the energy going up each of our chakras—not each with a separate body, but we are sharing the same chakras. Physically, we are one. Spiritually, we are one. We pull God upward into us

---

*There are several distinct "rings" of muscle within the vagina. Like fingers squeezing a rod, these muscles, when properly developed, can be individually controlled to massage the lingam.

from the earth as we move in slow, intense harmony, upward all the way through the crown chakra, the spiritual center, and outward. Now the energy of God rains down on us from the opposite direction, through the crown chakra and into our bodies.

With souls entwined, it feels as though God is inside us and outside us. The satiation is deeper than we thought possible. We have been seeking this moment of oneness since the day of birth and even before that. This is a healing of heart, a healing of separation, a healing of the myth of original sin. We feel God inside us. God is the energy now. God is each of us and both of us and God is our oneness. God is everything and nothing and in this moment we know the truth of his presence within our hearts as an eternal certainty. Radiating with love, we reach the highest peak of orgasm in a simultaneous instant of forever, and we know this single orgasm of us and God must echo throughout the universe.

As we lie in stillness, gently holding one another, I feel deeply connected to my partner. My heart feels full. I get a sense that I have found something that I have yearned for, for what seems like lifetimes, eternities; a sense of true spiritual connection. I breathe a deep sigh of relief. In this instant I know that I am never alone, nor have I ever been, nor will I ever be.

Lovers' Heart Meditation

It becomes easy to tap in to the perfection in our partners when we meditate on the hearts of our lovers. In this meditation we wish to feel what our partners are feeling. When done in unison, both partners will feel an incredible sense of oneness and fulfillment.

Within every spiritual path, the one thing that gives us the safety to open up, experience pain and tears and grief, and go beyond our inner hell is quite simply love. Love creates a sacred space, where we feel more and more safe to expose all of our hidden parts. No one can last on this path without love, for it pulls us through when we have not the strength to make it on our own.

I begin with my physical meditation (see page 71). Once my body is immersed in this pleasure, my mind is free to delve into the awareness of love. I focus on the wonderful relationship I have with my partner and on his intelligence, his sensitivity to my feelings, his great sense of humor. I visualize his physical heart as it pumps blood through his body. I see his heart chakra, which overlaps and surrounds his physical heart, the heart that is his soul. I go deep inside his soul's heart. I feel into it, see into it, and hear into it. I see its dimensions—it is vast. My whole body can fit inside his heart! I enter. There is plenty of room for me. His heart is soft and inviting and open. Now inside his heart, my unconditional love pours from my own heart and into his. I love everything within his heart, the parts that are pure light and the parts that are bruised and fragile. I am one with his heart, exactly as it is. I find the place within him that shines the brightest. I go inside this bright spot and send my love into it, so that it grows and expands and fills his heart. I feel this energy that is the creation of us, healing any pain he might have and increasing his joy a thousand times! I grow our hearts now to become as large as both of our physical bodies. Our bodies become infused with each other's love.

As we generate more and more sexual energy, I bring all of this energy upward into our hearts, so that everything transforms into pure love. Upon orgasm, I pull the entire physical experience up into our hearts.

Meditation of Bliss

This meditation has had a profound impact on my life outside tantra. Essentially it has taught me to retrain my emotions. My entire body has become the reference point for whatever I want to feel on an ongoing basis. When I train my body with pleasurable emotions, I take those emotions with me wherever I go.

In this meditation I attach physical pleasure to whatever positive emotion I want to fill my life with, such as happiness, self-confidence, love, peacefulness. My entire body becomes fused with the emotion, now fueled by the physical energy.

I begin the session as in the previous example, by first getting into a feeling of total pleasure through the physical awakening. We saturate our bodies in pleasure.

I concentrate on the emotion I wish to increase. On this day I choose self-confidence. In my mind's eye I go inside my partner's body to find his confidence. I discover it in his power chakra (the belly area). I now visualize inside my own body and find a small seed of confidence within my heart chakra. I visualize these two areas of us becoming larger. I see them merging together.

Once centered on this feeling of confidence, I then focus on the sexual energy between us. I take our combined power of confidence and feel it radiating within both of our root chakras. Our root chakras become the feeling of confidence. Once our root chakras are fully immersed in confidence, I see it rise into our sex chakras (the second chakras). Again, I infuse the confidence with the incredibly alive energy of our sexuality and fill our chakras with this great emotion. I continue with each chakra, all the way up to our crowns.

When it is time to climax, I see this emotion being pulled into the orgasm. The orgasm becomes the emotion.

Meditation on God

This meditation can be extremely healing for those of us who have issues around God and sexuality. In this meditation we will bring a physical manifestation of God into our lovemaking. Basically, we make love to God, who takes the form of a deity—for example, Jesus, Buddha, the Virgin Mary, Babaji.* If you can't think of any deity that inspires you, envision a god or goddess who is the physical form of God incarnate.

Once my body is thoroughly excited through the physical awakening meditation, in my mind's eye I visualize Babaji sitting inside my heart. I can see his whole body inside me. Looking very closely, I notice every aspect of him—his eyes, hair, lips, chest, legs. What he is wearing. If he is communicating with me. I feel his characteristics and personality. I know that he is pleased and flattered that I have invited him to be with us while we are making love. I feel his gratefulness to be with me. I feel his excitement to be with me.

---

*Babaji is a saint from the East who is said to have achieved physical immortality. He is somewhat the equivalent of Jesus in the West.

Now I bring him down into my root chakra. He blesses all the energy and pleasure that are contained within my root chakra. I feel him wanting me to have more energy and pleasure. I can feel him sending his own divine energy into this chakra. Now I bring this deity who enjoys and approves of me up into my sex chakra, and again I feel his essence radiating, charging this chakra with liquid gold. I continue to bring him up into all seven chakras, enjoying his presence in each part of me.

Now I feel this deity going into my partner. I visualize myself making love to this deity, this living image of God, and to my partner at the same time. Upon each orgasm, the three of us are taking part in this highest of pleasures. I see the deity achieve orgasm at the same time, sending increasing amounts of love into my partner's body and mine.

Infinite Orgasms 9

When finally my heart allowed me to venture inside, a thousand words could not describe what I next saw. Contained within this vast Center is not just the essence, the very substance of my heart: no, it is much more! Here resides the whole universe, everything, all that I see outside of myself plus all other planes of existence—it is All. It is the residence of Mother and Father God. And this is why the path of liberation begins, continues, and ends with the heart.

I felt a wave of joy and fell back into my lover's rhythmic slow embrace, let it take me on a ride. I felt into this center of my heart, pulled the sexual energies into this soft sweet infinite space, and when I orgasmed I felt an explosion, as though a star were exploding—so big I could not think of anything, I could not focus, I could only see flashes of huge white streaks of light, my body convulsing, my mind blank: yes, we are all made of stardust.

As I began to partake in the many joys of tantric meditation, my body became exceedingly sensitive to the subtle nuances of rhythm, rate, and pressure.

"Don't worry," my partner would say with a sparkle in his eye, "it gets better."

It gets better. And did it ever!

What constantly amazes me about tantra is that as extraordinary as the physical ecstasy may be, the real reward is in how incredibly peaceful, happy, and fulfilled I have become. These positive emotions fill my body with vitality and energy, even more than does the nectar of kundalini itself.

As we know, the key to tantra is in the building of the orgasm. We are never in any hurry in tantra; on the contrary, the objective is to delay the orgasm while increasing energy within the body. Yet the peak moment of sexual pleasure is the orgasm. Within tantra, this orgasm takes on an entirely new dimension.

I never in a million years would have thought that a simple orgasm could contain such intense subtlety and variety. The levels of orgasms are a continual, constant surprise to any student on this path. Below I share some of the orgasms that I have experienced through tantra. In order to impose some structure, I separate each type of orgasm so that it can be more easily defined. This does not do justice to the whole experience, of course, as a particular type of orgasm is rarely experienced in isolation. There may be times when I have several types at once, or all of them at once, or in a sequential order. There is absolutely no limit to the ways by which a human being can experience an orgasm.

External Orgasms

External orgasms are the most common and are characterized by muscle contractions of the particular region climaxing.

The external clitoral orgasm is the garden-variety sensation that we generally consider an "orgasm." This is caused by direct clitoral stimulation, be that through oral sex, intercourse, or manually. Most of the pleasure is felt at the center of the clitoris.

The clitoris is incredible. It has many special parts. One side of the clitoris can be brought to orgasm. The outside of its skin can be brought to orgasm. Its inside can be brought to orgasm. There are a thousand different ways to bring the clitoris to orgasm.

Every area of the yoni is capable of orgasm. The inner lips (labia minora), which cradle the opening of the yoni, can be brought to orgasm. The thick, larger outer lips (labia majora) can be brought to orgasm. *No stimulation to the clitoris is necessary to cause an orgasm.* Only the region that is reaching the climax needs to be stimulated.

Usually, one side of a woman's yoni is more sensitive than the other. The more sensitive side is the better side to start sensitizing and bringing to orgasm. Later, both sides can become very sensitive, but usually there will remain a more sensitive side. The orgasm will feel different for each side. Each side has a life of its own, with different needs and wants. It is very nice to bring the tantrika's outer and inner lips to orgasm before even touching the clitoris. When this happens, the clitoris becomes exceedingly sensitive. The clitoris is then a sumptuous dessert!

The two sides of the yoni correspond to the two channels of kundalini, which coil around the spine. Once kundalini is awakened, the side orgasm will produce kundalini flow up each of the corresponding channels. These two channels are known as *ida,* the female or yin (left) channel that flows upward and generally feels cool blue, and *pingala,* the male or yang (right) channel that receives energy from above and feels red/orange. It is good to balance the left and right sides by bringing both to the same number of orgasms.

The body's ability to achieve orgasm does not stop at the lips. By employing the same methods, we can just as easily sensitize the area outside the outer lips, where the legs and torso meet, and the inner thighs, all the way down to the feet! Also through the perineum and anus, and upward, above the clitoris, all the way up to the breasts—the entire body is capable of orgasm.

One day my partner surprised me as I lay on my stomach. Breathing very softly, his mouth in the shape of an O while soft warm heat poured from his mouth, he started at the base of my coccyx and gently slid the breath up my spine, his lips not even touching me, just his breath on my spine. Slowly he went up, and the small peach fuzz on my back seemed to stand on end, beckoning for more. It felt like an electric fire. Then he stopped at the back of my neck, and it was so stimulating that I actually had an orgasm in my neck!

The Butterfly's Kiss

So delicate is this orgasm that we have coined for it the word *butterfly*. Here my partner is licking so gently that my yoni seems to swell larger just so that it can rise up to meet his teasing tongue. He starts me at whatever pressure my yoni desires. Once I am very aroused, he begins to lick more and more lightly, but not so lightly that I lose concentration or interest. He maintains a balance between keeping me totally aroused, on that edge before orgasm, and moving his tongue ever more lightly.

When I achieve orgasm, a soft ecstasy ripples gently over my yoni. The clitoris, the inner lips, and the outer lips may all be involved, or sometimes it is just one of these areas. The orgasm lifts me high. I feel my body rise above me, as though I'm floating on a soft cloud. I feel spacey and light-headed.

Throbbing Orgasm

Convulsing, deep orgasms that ripple inside my clitoris, inside the vaginal walls, or outside on my lips feel as primal as the beating of drums. The best time for this type of orgasm is toward the end of foreplay. Generally the throbbing orgasm is produced from steady licking combined with a strong focus on sending energy into the yoni. The throbbing orgasm is grounding, causing me to desire intensely the pleasure of the lingam. This is the type of orgasm that makes me moan with pleasure.

Extended Orgasms

It is possible for the body to maintain orgasm for two, five, thirty, and sixty minutes at a stretch. It will take time to build up to this long. The sex organ is a like a muscle: it grows with usage.

Retaining extended orgasms is as much psychological as it is physical. We need to know that we deserve pleasure. When my orgasms initially began to lengthen, I noticed that it was my mind first, not my body, that said, "Okay, that's enough pleasure. Time to stop." And then my body would shut down. I believe the body is capable of maintaining a constant state of orgasm. This will take years of practice. Let us begin by first lengthening the pleasure that we already know. Over the years our personal threshold of pleasure will rise. There is no rush. In tantra, there is never a need to rush.

Internal Orgasms

Internal orgasms are brought about by the same stimulation as external orgasms, but they actually travel inside the body. There are no contractions or outward sensations. As with an external orgasm, it feels as though I am dropping off a cliff and totally letting go. But here there is no external experience, and instead of sensations of physical pleasure there is silence. Internal orgasms typically happen prior to external orgasms, as a setup to the external orgasm. These can also happen during very slow oral sex. All I feel is the beating of my heart, my blood flowing. And then I feel a certain energy leading upward, pulled by the flow of blood. All energy is brought inward and upward.

Internal orgasms can be anticlimactic, even frustrating. This is because I'm brought over the edge into the orgasmic state, but instead of this loud release, the outer pleasure withdraws inward, and I feel just this silence combined with a pounding heart.

Internal orgasms are good for us because they direct our sexual energy up inside the body. In a sense the body becomes lubricated with energy. This energy keeps us vibrant and young. A recent study in Britain linked the frequency of orgasms to lowering the average mortality rate, concluding that sexual activity seems to have a protective effect on one's health.* Imagine now that we are taking all the health-producing effects of orgasms and bringing them inward. Internal orgasms will arouse dormant kundalini. The stillness allows our minds to become keenly focused on meditative experience.

G-spot Orgasms

The G-spot, located about two inches inside the vaginal canal and on the anterior of the body, is most commonly stimulated by the lingam. Men and women do fit together like a hand in a glove!

*Davey G. Smith, "Sex and Death: Are They Related? Findings from the Caerphilly Cohort Study," *British Medical Journal,* 20 December 1997: 1641–44.

G-spot orgasms vary just as do external orgasms. Some will feel decentralized, throughout the whole body. Some will be accompanied by pelvic convulsions.

My partner and I experiment with different sexual positions to find which ones stimulate both of us the most. Again, however, I find that less is more. Pounding friction is not the goal here. The idea is to have the maximum amount of arousal with the least amount of stimulation. We may stay inside each other with almost no movement whatsoever except for the squeezing of my vaginal muscles. A goal—which I have not yet mastered— is when a woman can bring a man to orgasm just with the contraction of her vaginal muscles.

The wonderful thing about G-spot orgasms is the intimacy we feel with our partners. There is no greater physical closeness than when a man is physically inside a woman, the two breathing together, hearts open and minds at one. When a woman achieves orgasms in this state, with a man holding her close, it is like finding completion. When we climax with our partners simultaneously, the pleasure is exponential.

Chakra Orgasms

When we have finally mastered inner and outer orgasms, the orgasms rise to fill our entire bodies. Every part and particle of us will begin to experience each orgasm. We will experience an orgasm inside each chakra. We will have an orgasm in our power centers, then in the heart chakra, then in the throat chakra.

Once we get to the higher levels of the third eye and crown chakra, the orgasm will be exceptionally strong, even disorienting. It is not uncommon to feel spacey and light-headed for a long time after the orgasm. This type of orgasm might feel very odd, but it will not harm us. It will bring much joy, for with orgasms of this kind we are opening more of ourselves.

Spiritual Orgasms

Once we master orgasms in each chakra, we are ready for the next level: the spiritual orgasm. A spiritual orgasm occurs outside the body. In the beginning the orgasm will seem to take place six to eight inches above the head. It feels as though this orgasm, above the head, is pulling the whole body up into it! This is a very advanced level of orgasm. We will have pushed ourselves beyond what our physical body can contain on its own. This is a major step in the journey to spiritual oneness with all others. At this point we must remain focused on the love we have found within us, and take it with us into the orgasm. Our love is the glue that binds us with another's spirit. The concept of an outer orgasm will take on a whole new meaning, as it involves all of us and beyond. But a spiritual orgasm is not the goal. It is just a tool to help bring us to oneness with our spiritual selves, with others, and with God.

The body, a microcosm of human nature, loves patterns. My partner has developed a pattern of stimulating me that I have really become quite attached to. He starts at my inner thighs and then travels inward very, very slowly. He might bring my right outer lip to orgasm first and then the outer left lip, and then travels inward, and so forth. Because of this pattern, which is the result of combining my personal desires with his incredible skills, I have run into some challenges with other lovers. You see, it takes time for lovers to understand each other's patterns. My tantric partner knows me so well that he has set a very high standard for my boyfriends. I have had experiences in which I was making love to my boyfriend but wanting him to do exactly what my tantric partner does to me. Of course, I know it isn't fair to compare one man to another.

I had yet to discover how to integrate the seemingly fragmented parts of my life.

Personality
Transformation

e lifts my body nearer to climax and suddenly I am somewhere else, somewhere in the clouds, somewhere not on Earth, that is certain. And here is where the energy seems to take my mind on a ride, and now is when I can think of nothing. Now is when I can only feel, and certain images and memories arise, and all of it is being controlled by the energy. Oh God, he takes me into climax, and I follow along.

A memory comes into me, this memory long forgotten, a dream from childhood, a recurring dream I used to have where my body would feel almost like mud, as though the parts of me, the physical and soul parts of me, are morphing, enlarging and shrinking—I slip into this vivid remembrance as I am orgasming and strangely feel a sense of completion and rightness and transcendence.

A big part of following any spiritual path is learning lessons. These lessons are designed to help us realize our highest potential. Typically this asks for us to refine our characters. Religions vary greatly in their definition of human refinement and can be recognized based on how that refinement is brought about. Some religions mandate actions. Orthodox Judaism governs the strict details of kosher eating in order to adhere to holy laws. Jehovah's Witnesses seek to convert others to their faith.

Whether or not we agree on the means, the unifying message is to transform ourselves to become better. Simply put, we can change. We have innate physiological triggers for major life changes, also known as rites of passage (puberty and menopause are examples). These transformations are difficult. But to want to change beyond these basic rites is what many find impossible. It is not so easy to change, let alone have the desire. As functioning, healthy adults, why should we bother changing anything at all?

We like things the way they are. Even when we know that change will make us happier and more fulfilled, we fear change. It is human nature to preserve itself. We all have an ego, whose very reason for existence is our survival. The ego perceives change as negative because change threatens our sense of survival. The ego justifies this primitive urge with very real feelings of fear, self-doubt, and anger. The ego is stubborn and always has an undercurrent of rebellion; ultimately, the rebellion is against God. Negative emotions always hold us back.

Yet also pulling at our conscience is the nature of humankind to grow. Our souls call on us to become better, and we know this in the stillest and deepest part of the mind. We feel something inside of us that is bigger than ourselves, something that connects us to a greater purpose.

And so we feel this pull between the ego's desire to stay the same and the soul's desire to become better. To some extent, we will always have this dichotomy within us. But all is not hopeless. We can teach the ego to serve our highest good, and we can teach ourselves to listen to the calling of the soul.

There came a point when I had moved forward so much—getting rid of my issues around sex, improving my ability to empathize and to get along with others, becoming more present in intimate situations—that I hit a wall. It was as though my ego was allowing me to let go of only some small issues so that certain areas of my life would improve. But then I began to feel a lot of resistance to change. The next level would be more than making small improvements. The next level would be a major shift for me.

Transformation within tantra is, like all of tantra, practical. In tantra the perception is that we will find true inner happiness by transforming our personalities. We transform our personalities in a very efficient way: through mastering our emotions.

Because emotions bind together our personalities, they are the ideal place to start. We respect our emotions and defend them valiantly. Indeed, we think we are our emotions. Look back on an important event in your childhood. What is it that you remember? Is it not the pervading emotion, whether joy, humiliation, or sorrow? When the facts fade away, emotions are the memories we keep. Emotions are what we bring to consciousness as we fall asleep in the evening and as we awaken each morning. We identify who we are with our emotions. We believe they are what make up *us*.

Our sexuality is tied tightly to our sense of identity, and hence our emotions. Have you ever cried during or right after lovemaking, for no apparent reason? Have you ever felt a moment of intense fear as a stabbing throb right in the center of your genitals, even though the fear had nothing to do with sex? Sexuality seems to fuse with our deepest feelings, good and bad, from rapturous joy to the urge for death.

But we are not our emotions. We only *feel* that we are. Similarly, we only think we are our personality. In truth, our personalities and our emotions are a veil of illusion; a cloak of our true identities. It is easy to recognize this with the example of an unruly, impetuous young boy who grows up to be a sweet and lovely man. This man is nothing like he was as a boy, yet the boy, at the age of seven, believes he knows who he is. Over the course of life, our emotional and perceptional contexts can change completely, often more than once (although, admittedly, some people never change). Even though our emotional characters change, and our personalitiesy metamorphose, at all times we are who we are. We are always our essence. We are always spirit.

Our emotions are a good and necessary part of human nature. The question is whether we let our emotions dictate to us or whether we consciously choose them. The world around us often operates on the former principle— to let our emotions run free. Film often promotes heroes who act on passions, giving us role models who benefit when they give in to emotion. Advertisements appeal to our emotions, beseeching us to submit to that driving part of our ego. Some of the self-help movement focuses on expressing emotions; primal scream therapy is an extreme example.

The media also show the opposite: adolescent gang members kill innocent victims in a drive-by shooting, or teenagers shoot their schoolmates in the classroom. These situations are acute and tragic examples of people giving in to their emotions. Some believe that we are approaching a national epidemic of this kind in both small towns and large cities. We must remember what the term *civilized* is supposed to mean: it means having a certain amount of respect for others, and often this means controlling our emotions by watching what we say and what we do to others. Increasing our emotional energy without having control over our emotions can lead to catastrophic problems within society. Hitler knew this power when he whipped crowds into a patriotic frenzy by playing on their emotions.

Ironically, we learn at a young age to suppress our emotions. Our truth might make others feel uncomfortable. A child's unedited extremes of happiness and sadness, joy and upset, might trigger an adult's fear of his or her own emotions. So in one regard we are taught not to feel and at the same time blindly to follow our emotions without regard to logic. But these extremes are the opposite side of the same coin. Both extremes allow us to remain unaware of how much our emotions are really controlling us.

One way to overcome being a slave to our emotions is abstaining from that which typically induces emotional attachments such as material possessions, personal relationships, and sex. The monastery, for instance, creates such an environment. The idea is to see through the temporality of emotions and in so doing, to realize who we really are beyond the surface clutter of the mind. Sex, of course, is something that we can be very attached to—it's the life-sustaining tool of humanity. But the objective of tantra is exactly the same as a path of abstinence. Tantra uses sexual energy to transcend our mundane attachments to sex. Similarly, Tantra embraces our emotions so that they serve to assist our enlightenment. Our emotions become the catalyst for transformation.

Transcending emotions does not mean that once we become enlightened we magically cease to feel anything. The concept is that at the core of our nature, we are pure joy. The negative simply goes away—because that is not who we really are. The positive remains, and keeps getting better. Positive emotions are the expression of who we really are. Just as our desire for sex is transformed into spiritual desire, so all of our negativity is transformed into positivity.

This concept initially confused me. How can you have white without black, day without night, joy without sorrow? In our world, we are able to perceive mainly because things have opposites.

My partner explained to me one day in a metaphor. "Can you see a white dot against a white background?" he asked.

"Of course not," I replied. "That's what I'm saying!"

"Does the fact that you can't see the dot against the white background mean that it doesn't exist?"

That made me think. When we can look objectively at our emotions without attachment, there is a profound sense of freedom. We are no longer tied to these chains that seem to control our happiness. We may accept this argument intellectually. Self-control and happiness are good things, after all. But tantra has no interest in philosophical acceptance, nor in metaphors about white dots.

I can still remember the moment that this clicked. That day I finally understood that the path was about *changing myself*, or at least who I thought I was, in order to become truly happy. Changing not just my views about sex, or some surface emotional problems, but myself—huge chunks of my personality. The things that made me tick. The *emotional* me. Mind you, this was not for several years into my study of tantra. It's easy to know something without walking the talk!

I must change my emotions?

And there is no way around this?

But shouldn't I be the one exception to this rule?

But I'm perfect! screamed my guts.

I was not afraid of how difficult it might be to change. I was not paralyzed by fear of the unknown. The real issue was that I had now become aware of my unconscious agenda. I had expected the tantric path to change to suit me, Valerie Brooks. I had expected my salvation simply to arrive once I announced: "I am on a spiritual path." I had this picture that my tantric path would shower me with gifts and great happiness. I had not made the connection that great happiness might require me to change.

Religion is famous for placating masses of people who hold the same beliefs that I did. How else can we explain the centuries of societies that have shuffled off to worship every Sabbath and yet continue the cycles of war, cruelty, and hatred? It comes from the idea that we do not need to change ourselves, that as long as we do certain things, we will be saved, and our righteousness puts us above the rules, unaccountable for harming others.

We blame God for the cruelty in the world, yet is not most of this cruelty done by our own hands?

True growth stems from responsibility. Instead of preaching about love and peace, we must live these principles. This does not come naturally. We must consciously uncover each dark corner of the mind, which hates, covets, and fears.

I must start by changing myself. I must stop blaming. I must stop waiting for the world around me to fix itself. Any time I expect or want something outside of myself to save or fix me, I must realize how ridiculous I am being. Personal responsibility, I realized, is the key to personality transformation.

On the day that I really digested and accepted this truth, I suffered a massive headache. But from that day forward, things that had seemed difficult got a lot easier. If all I must do is work to change and improve my own personality, my life would be so much simpler. And my happiness—might I even say the happiness of the world—was in my own hands, within my reach!

But first, because I'm more stubborn than a brick wall, I needed proof. I needed to experience whether my emotions were *not me*. Second, I had to find out whether it would be in my best interest to change.

Emotional memories are not stored just in the brain; they are deeply embedded in the body. There is an increasing amount of evidence that points to the idea that the body, not only the mind, holds emotional memories. Among these are the Rosen Method, founded by psychotherapist Marion Rosen. The rebirthing movement also adopts this principle, as do some theories of physical massage, Rolfing, and other types of bodywork. Being so physical in nature, tantra naturally pushes up unconscious or suppressed emotions to the surface of the conscious mind very quickly.

As a freshly developing tantrika and a passionately emotional woman, I decided to embark on my research experiment on whether I should change my emotions with the most obvious and intriguing of first choices: sex. I thought I had fixed my issues about sex through tantric meditation. When I practiced tantra, it had stirred up these feelings inside me about sex being wrong. *Sex is not something God wants me to feel good about. Sex is dirty. Sex is evil.* To my adult conscious self, I knew these thoughts were ridiculous. Tantric meditation did not work only to heal these emotions, but also led me to my subconscious feelings that lay underneath these views.

The issue I thought I had was not what I was really upset about. *Sex is bad*—this is a *surface* emotion. As I accepted my surface emotions, like the skins of an onion they would slowly fall aside to reveal the meat—true emotions driving me. I had to look for what was not so obvious.

It is easy to identify which layer of emotion we are consciously aware of. Surface emotions generally involve feelings about something outside ourselves—another person or event, for example—over which we seemingly have no control. Surface emotions can appear to an objective outsider as blown out of proportion. They often involve anger or blame. *Inner* emotions, on the other hand, become increasingly personal, having nothing whatsoever do with anything but our own actions, and then even deeper, our own feelings about ourselves.

I knew I had to go deeper because I was relating to sex, which was happening to me. So forget about everything that is external to me. How did I feel about my own sexuality?

I practiced my tantra as usual, but in our few minutes of prayer before we started tantra, I would ask to know my subconscious emotions more deeply.

As a sexual woman, I am valuable because I am a giver of life. I can create a child. My sexuality is a powerful creative force. My sexuality is a power that makes me desirable and attractive to others. My sexuality is intense, and vibrant, and the more tantra I do, the more powerful and full of life energy I feel!

But looking deeper, I discovered a fear, hidden deep within my gut, that sexuality takes away my power and value. I am not valued *because* I am a woman, and women have less power in this world. I am not truly valued because I am seen only as a sex object. If I am a woman who is sexual, I am a whore, a slut, and a sinner. If I enjoy sex, I am even *more* slutty, wrong, and sinful. In fact, the more I enjoy sexual pleasure, the more monstrous and ugly I become! My sexuality is shameful and wrong, and I chose tantra because I am wrong.

Notice the last word in the above paragraph. The whole exploration of sex and my sexuality ultimately had nothing to do with sex. It had to do with a much simpler, much more basic issue: me. My relationship with myself. I felt wrong.

The deepest layer of any emotional issue has to do with very simple, very personal feelings, or *root* emotions. Root emotions develop during the first few years of life and unconsciously pervade much of our sense of identity. These have also been called personal laws or, more appropriately, personal *lies*.* Most people have three root emotions, and at least one of them will underlie nearly all negative feelings. Root emotions are simple "I" statements such as *I am bad, I'm unwanted, I don't exist, I can't*, and *I'm not good enough*. My root emotion that *I am wrong* had sunk so deeply that it hurt to look at it even for a moment.

Facing root emotions is not something our conscious mind wants to do, because it is difficult and unpleasant. I had felt wrong about things before. But I had never consciously acknowledged that this feeling of wrongness was mired in the depth of my soul. It was so pervading that it felt like who I am.

My mind wanted to think of anything but this. I wanted to run away and bury my head in the sand. But taking a deep breath, I focused on where this wrongness was in my body—I felt it inside my stomach, a black, sickly wrongness burning in my belly. I sank into the feeling. At that moment the pain suddenly eased. Sometimes just becoming conscious of root emotions will help to heal them.

I had a big case of low self-esteem. All the pain and fear about sex—about anything in my life, for that matter—came back to my not feeling good about myself.

I didn't know how to get from feeling intrinsically wrong to feeling intrinsically good about myself. But I was so unhappy that I knew I needed some sort of change. And somewhere, calling out from deep within me, I just knew that my wrongness was not me.

In that moment I realized that the fundamental *I* was neither set of emotions. I had a choice as to which to keep and which to discard. And you can guess which ones I wanted to get rid of.

At the innermost core of all negative thoughts is one ultimate lie. This lie is simple, but it is the basis of human suffering. The ultimate lie is that we are separate from God. Believing we are separate is where the whole

---

*Authors Leonard Orr and Sondra Ray are credited with coining the term *personal lies*. Any book written by these revolutionary thinkers is highly recommended.

concept of original sin was born. Feeling separate from God is the illusion of the world that we are all here to overcome. Of course this lie is not true. But the key is to embody the truth that we are one with God. The healing of all negative emotions, small and large, leads us toward healing the lie that we are separate from God.

Emotions and Kundalini

Time revealed many lessons to help me deal with my emotions. Some were dramatic, such as my personal lie of "I am wrong"—this core issue did not disappear overnight. It would come up, incident by incident, and each time I had to recognize it for what it was.

The increasing kundalini in my body sped up the process of my emotional healing. It did not let me get away with as much, especially my anger. Kundalini can awaken once we have attained a certain amount of personal mastery. Sometimes, however, it can awaken beyond our current level of spiritual enlightenment, and therefore, for a period of time, our physical bodies may be more "evolved" than our minds.

When I first began to experience my aroused kundalini, I was enamored with it. Oh yes, I thought I was pretty wonderful! Wow, I must be really spiritual if I'm getting this kundalini already! Any tool, even a spiritual tool such as kundalini, can be used to advance the motives of the ego. In fact, spiritual tools are especially suspect because they seem so well justified. After all, I did a great deal of tantra to produce this result within my body!

But that was just my ego playing its usual games of superiority. And my arrogance soon came to a halt. For weeks I had been intensely practicing tantra. At the same time, I was working hard at my job as a sales executive for a software firm. It was just after the end of the fiscal year, and I had worked serious overtime to close several important deals. This fateful morning, when I received my commission statement, I discovered that my company had grossly miscalculated what I was owed, and I had reason to believe it was intentional. As the day progressed, my tantric high lingered inside my body while my conscious mind tackled this startling problem. Although my body felt great from the kundalini, I became more and more furious as time went on! No one would acknowledge that there was a problem, and my boss was definitely avoiding me. I felt victimized and cheated. Normally I would simply stew in anger and hold my fire until I could correct things. The difference on this day was that every time I felt a wave of anger, I began to feel increasingly nauseous. The more I dwelled on my upset, the more I wanted to throw up. It felt as though my physical body was repulsed by my own negative emotions.

The physiological effects of anger came in contact with my kundalini, and it was like a struggle between good and evil. Both hated having the other there, but the kundalini was the stronger party. So here I was, caught in the middle of this physical tumult, feeling as though my stomach was turning inside out, getting hot flashes and headaches. The physical pain began to feel worse than my commission problem, worse than my anger.

After repeated episodes to the rest room to relieve the nausea, I realized how foolish I had been. I could hear this voice in my head saying, *"The kundalini is there for a reason, Valerie!"* My kundalini was there to help me become more enlightened, and my feelings of anger and rage were no longer appropriate responses. My body was beginning to reject these emotions, and it was high time that I took responsibility and consciously chose to let go of more of my negative emotions. *My body was becoming my teacher.*

That day, I chose to let go of my anger. I chose physical health and emotional well-being over negative emotions. Only then did the pain within my body subside. (Incidentally, the commission issue was quickly fixed the moment my manager had a chance. I could be just as powerful without needing to get angry.)

My anger was a surface emotion. What lay beneath it? Again, *I am wrong.* My anger was an attempt to prove to the company that I was right! It's amazing how these root emotions keep appearing.

But kundalini does not care if I am right or wrong. It prefers that I be happy.

Facing one's dark sides comes up over and over in spiritual teachings. In *The Path: A Spiritual Autobiography* by J. Donald Walters, the author describes how his teacher and yoga master, Paramahansa Yogananda, undergoes an intensive spiritual retreat into the woods, where, contrary to experiencing bliss and happiness, he faces the most unpleasant facets of himself, his ugliest and darkest sides.* In Western religion we see this also: Jesus goes into the desert for forty days and nights to face his inner demons. He was dealing with the devil inside him. Kundalini awakens our highest level of conscience and integrity, which will naturally lead us to emotional healing and spiritual integrity—not by indoctrination, but by personal choice.

Tantra, however, was not the magic bullet that would solve all my problems. I would need other disciplines to help direct and balance this immense energy inside me.

---

* J. Donald Walters, *The Path: A Spiritual Autobiography* (Nevada City, Calif.: Ananda Publications, 1977).

Balancing 11
Tantra

*M*y chakras are on fire, open, impassioned, *throbbing. I envisioned God supporting me from behind, as though I lay on top of him, and his hands reached through me and held my heart to this infinite cascade of light that poured from the heavens into me. I felt warm liquid pour out from my coccyx and up into God's hands. My energy today feels balanced and strong. It feels like am with God.*

All emotions are intensified through the use of tantra: both the negative and the positive. The more tantra I practiced, the more I understood why I had needed to spend two years first learning and practicing other disciplines that would help me to direct the energy from tantra.*

Human beings have a penchant for misery and suffering. We bask in it, as though unhappiness is what keeps us alive. Many artists believe that creative inspiration comes from human suffering. When we let ourselves experience higher and higher doses of pleasure, we will feel parts of ourselves begging to remain negative.

* In *Highest Yoga Tantra*, Daniel Cozort explains the nineteenth-century tantric text "Illumination of the Texts of Tantra," which describes the steps of tantra. Interestingly, the first half of the disciplines described refer only to meditation, with no tantric sex whatsoever (New York: Snow Lion Publications, 1986).

The pleasure spectrum (see chapter 7) operates in the same way as does our emotional spectrum. We let ourselves experience a range between happiness and suffering, love and hate, control and surrender. Most people are accustomed to being unhappy and stressed most of the time. We are drama queens and kings! What we know as reality is the subjective collection of incidents that we allow ourselves to experience. Expand the spectrum, and we will change our realities.

Our emotional selves need time to adjust to a new context of feeling good. Negative emotions that are accustomed to their place in our minds and bodies will want their turn! Our bodies are addicted to our emotional patterns. When we feel anger, worry, upset, or fear, hormones are released into the bloodstream. We get doses of emotional hormone all day long. Thus, we will find our negative emotions begging for attention more than ever.

It was more difficult than you can imagine for me to accept the constantly increasing, almost unearthly levels of pleasure that are the side effects of tantra. I had to learn that happiness was not going to hurt me.

In prayer we speak to God, and in meditation we listen to God. Meditation allows us to stabilize ourselves, to clear the clutter of our minds so that God's direction may become more evident. All life is blessed with consciousness. But human cognition, our ability to reason, is what sets us apart from our raw emotions, from the animal kingdom.

But frankly, I hated meditation.

It seemed that sitting in stillness and eliminating all distractions would be boring and unimportant compared to tantra. When I began to meditate, however, I soon realized that what I really disliked was the fact that meditation forced me to choose between my (ego) thoughts and higher thoughts. It caused me to admit that all the mind chatter running pell-mell through my consciousness was of little value.

If you're one of those rare individuals talented with the natural ability to enjoy the stillness of mind, you're very fortunate. I practically had to force myself to meditate. I tried an inner rhythm method in which I would meditate just when I felt like it. That failed miserably. Evening meditation didn't work for me because I could always find something better to do. Then I figured that because I had so much resistance, I must need more meditation than did other people, so I set up a regimen of three hours per day. That

experiment never even saw the light of day! The last attempt finally stuck—
every morning, thirty minutes a day. That way, I reasoned, I could get it over
with quickly! Yet as time went on, I grew to love and need my meditation so
much that now I not only look forward to each morning of solitude, but
occasionally also extend the thirty minutes to an hour. If we can meditate
for thirty minutes three times a week, plus practice tantra, we will achieve
very impressive results.

There are many great books available on the subject of meditation, and I
will not attempt to go into the level of detail that you will need. However,
let me generally describe the process. There are two types of focus during
meditation:

1. Focus on one thing, to the exclusion of everything else.
2. Focus on nothing.

Generally, the first will result in the second. That is usually the easiest way.
The three types of focused meditation are as follows:

1. Mandala Focus. Focus on an object inside the mind's eye, often
   highly detailed, to the exclusion of all else.
2. Mantra Focus. Focus consciousness on inner sound—that is,
   sound heard not with the ear but with the mind.
3. Physical Focus. Doing moving meditations, during which one
   is physically involved in dancing, chanting, or deliberate
   movement.

The purpose of each is the same, which is to absorb the mind, body, and
emotions to the point where all mundane, ego-based thoughts are transcended. In this state the mind becomes a channel for higher intelligence.
We learn to listen to God.

Meditation reversed a desperately bad habit that had burdened me like
thousand-pound weights on my shoulders. This habit was worry. I worried
about everything! My mind spinned in a million directions over every possible problem, both real and imaginary. I worried about the future and the
past. I worried about what people said and about what they didn't say. I
worried about my flaws and my talents. Nothing escaped my worry radar.

But worry was tied to my sense of self-doubt. When I meditated, I had to set aside all personal issues. I learned that all my criticizing self-doubt, however real it felt, was little more than droning, useless mind chatter. Like all emotions, it was simply a pattern I had developed. As I learned to objectify myself from my worrisome "problems," I began to see that for every problem there are many solutions.

In the stillness of my mind, after I do a focused meditation, I focus on nothing. I am listening, and it is at this time that my best ideas and solutions appear from nowhere, effortlessly. The lightbulb goes on.

I also found that I could help others in this same way. When I was in the real world, going about my day, I would take the concern of someone and project my mind's eye into the other person's stillness inside him or her. I could mentally go inside that person's own inspiration, as it were, and tune in to the solution that lay inside of his own mind. People began to regard me as more of a leader who could provide suggestions to help.

Not bad for boring old meditation!

Tantric meditation uses a combination of these basic techniques. (Nothing new has been invented!) We focus on the body to the exclusion of all else. We incorporate mantra through the playing of music and mandala by focusing on our partners' hearts (as one example), and the physical expression is the sexual act. There comes a point when the mind goes into a void. Usually for me that will be after the first orgasm, and thereafter, depending on the situation, my focus will go in and out of this state.

Emotion as Energy

One day my partner taught me an extremely powerful technique to transform emotion. Emotions are nothing but energy. When tantra brings up emotions that I do not wish to hold on to, I can see the emotion as pure energy and then direct it to what I want to feel instead. I can use the energy to increase the opposing emotion.

The first step was for me to learn how to approach all negative emotions from a place of neutrality: saying each time, "Good, I accept this emotion. I am glad I feel this emotion." I welcome the emotion into my body, letting it be there, letting it be okay. This works well for any feeling: anger, jealousy, insecurity, sadness.

As I begin to accept this emotion, the feeling comes on really strong, like a raging river finally overflowing its banks. The feeling has been suppressed for so long that it wants its turn! This burst of emotion lasts only a few minutes, and sometimes not even that long. As the feeling rushes to the surface, I sit quietly and continue to say, *I accept and welcome this feeling.* Very quickly, the emotion will become significantly neutralized. Sometimes an emotion just wants attention, like a child. Often, just being fully conscious of a feeling is half the battle.

The next step is to transform the emotion by using the emotion's energy to become its opposite. In other words, I use my sadness to feel happy. I use my insecurity to feel confident. I use my jealousy to feel generous. I use my anger to feel forgiveness.

When I discovered my feeling of wrongness, I said, "Good, I accept that my sexuality is wrong. I'm glad I'm wrong as a sexual woman. I'm glad I'm wrong. Every time I feel wrong, I will use this feeling to feel good and right."

Transforming negative emotion into its positive counterpart feels strange at first. It will not change the negative emotion overnight. The sequence of the affirmation—first acceptance, then transformation—must be repeated whenever that negative feeling comes up. In my case, I felt a sense of acute wrongness for weeks after my discovery, and every time I felt it I had to force myself to say the above affirmation, with conviction in both my heart and my voice. But eventually my mind had nothing else to do but to obey my wishes. I was not suppressing the emotion, but I was giving my mind something to do with it. The mind always wants something to do. We cannot simply take away our negative emotions—we must replace them with something else.

Other types of meditation that I have used in conjunction with tantra are as follows:

- Prayer: life becomes more tranquil when we let God help us
- Fasting: important for cleansing the body, mind, and spirit
- Rebirthing (conscious breathing): to tap quickly into root emotions

- Cobra breath: opens the third eye and raises kundalini*
- Kriya yoga: a path that combines disciplined, meditative breathing with a life of rightful action

Our personalities are really nothing more than a complex set of habits, or patterns. Through tantric meditation, combined with the above disciplines, we uncover these many complex patterns, one small piece at a time. We learn to surrender to these patterns by becoming one with them. We let go of the patterns that do not serve us, and we enhance the patterns that serve our highest good.

We walk a balance between surrender and creation.

As we address more and more of the smaller patterns, we will notice that large parts of ourselves will shift. We begin the process of personality transformation. We start consciously transforming who we are. We can change our destinies. We can alter karma.

But because we do not live inside a vacuum, at some point we will need to go farther. How does mastery of the inner world relate to the external world, beyond the barriers of our own skin and minds?

---

*The cobra breath is an eight-step system of kriya yoga that must be learned through a teacher who is authorized as an initiator. As a student, I cannot reveal the details of the cobra breath, because its effectiveness lies in the fact that it must be given orally only from teacher to student. The cobra breath can be practiced both in private and during tantra.

Beyond Emotions 12

*t*he goddess of sexuality transforms my body into a temple
*occupied by herself, by a light, a blue-green cool and red-orange hot that
courses through and feels like water and fire tickling my cells, licking
me deeply. I become the icon of female transcendence. I am she who has
risen from the ashes with red-hot flowing hair like uncoiled serpents. I
am transcended beyond mundane reality, beyond illusion, beyond all that
is trapped in time. I ride this wave, I ride this goddess, and this goddess
mounts me and then we are both one, both coming together—we are all,
we are opposites combined. We are joy and despair, we are life and death,
we are one with all that is, we are vibrant body and weightless spirit.*

Once we master our own patterns, we can begin to discover the patterns of
the world outside our own flesh. These are what we call external patterns.
We discover *external patterns* in much the same way as we address our own
selves. We must first become one with them.

Nearly every aspect of our lives relates to the world around us. I can
meditate all I want, but once I step outside my home and begin to interact
with others in the world, I must deal with real life. In tantra we do not have
this exemption; even meditation is done with others.

The first step to understanding external patterns is being aware of the
present moment. This becomes much easier once we clear up a large portion

of our personal emotional negativity. When we feel positive and in balance, we become clear conduits for what is presently happening, instead of imposing our personal issues onto things.

When we are one with the patterns of the world outside us, we can become part of the conscious creation process of the universe. We are already a part of the cosmic dance; our mere existence proves that this is so. It is impossible *not* to affect the world around us. But so much of what we do is not conscious.

Everything in our lives is based on patterns: from brushing our teeth, to the problems we encounter again and again in our relationships. In order to master outer patterns, we turn to the faithful teacher, the tantric partner. We learn to master our partners' physical patterns by, of course, becoming one during the sexual act. We learn to listen to everything our partners want and need. We can train our partners to become increasingly more orgasmic. This is where the bodies of two will meld into one, for it becomes blurry who is leading and who is following. Once I am one with my partner, I can guide him to becoming more ecstatic, happier, and more in love.

The physical world is ruled by patterns (even chaotic models prove this).* Sunrise and sunset, the cycles of the Moon, the four seasons, and the rotation of Earth: all follow obvious patterns. Just as our emotions are a shadow of everlasting joy, the patterns of Earth are a reflection of the deeper patterns of the universe that we cannot so easily see with the naked eye. In physics, patterns of the universe become so specific and predictable that they can be mathematically calculated.

When I was nineteen I was like many college students in that I had to support myself. I worked very, very hard, for I believed that the only thing that would get me anywhere in the world was to throw myself into my work—both school and job. I kept pushing, burning the midnight oil, never stopping. Then I wondered why I was still having so many financial problems. You may argue that it had to do with my youth and inexperience in the workplace. But this was not the case. At one point I had three separate jobs!

---

*In *Chaos Theory Tamed* by Garrett P. Williams (National Academy Press, 1997), the author describes that all chaos eventually produces stable, repeatable patterns.

Yes, it had to do with my youth, but only because I had not gained the wisdom of understanding outer patterns.

The Bible says: "To every thing there is a season, and a time to every purpose under heaven" (Ecclesiastes). In order to master money, I had to learn its patterns. We are in relationship with everything around us. Money is a relationship. The one part about money that I had not learned was when to listen to it. I certainly talked to money a lot—I was always pushing to get it. Yet just as in meditation, when we listen to God and receive our long-awaited answers, so I had to learn when to listen to money. I had to learn when money was asking me simply to hold out my hands and encompass the opportunity that was right in front of me.

I discovered that like the physical body, which has patterns that must be mastered by both our partners and ourselves, money has patterns that must be mastered by listening, watching, taking action when appropriate, and allowing ourselves to receive when the time arises. When I finally began to understand the patterns of money, my financial problems disappeared.

In the span of only a few years my relationship with money shifted from being bad to okay, then from okay to good, then from good to great, then from great to incredible. I have achieved a level of financial success for which I am extremely grateful. It has given me the freedom to let go of struggle and focus on the things that are really important in life, such as my spiritual self. Having financial independence helps me relax.

More interesting was my resistance to giving up my poverty, for money makes a great excuse. After all, if I'm poor, I can't possibly have the time to pursue diligently my spiritual path, improve my relationships with friends and family, or work on my personal development. I have more practical things to do. Poverty is also the reflection that life must be a struggle. And I loved to struggle! But knowing that I had these reasons for wanting to keep prosperity out of my life helped me realize why I had money problems in the first place. There is a saying that whatever is happening in our lives is exactly what we want.

At work, I also learned how to master the patterns of my prospective customers. Just as I was learning, through meditation both during and outside of tantra, to look more deeply into myself and uncover more layers of truth, so I learned how to apply this skill toward others. As a sales executive

I was given ample opportunity to understand the patterns of others. I began to listen to what was not being said, to see what they felt in their hearts but were not verbalizing. I learned how to ask the right questions so that I could understand what made them tick, and what made the company tick. In so doing, I reached a level of empathy that allowed me to become one with them, and to be on their side, as opposed to me selling on the other side of the table. It was not about "me against them." In so caring for what they really wanted and needed, the prospective customers and I would quickly decide together whether I could offer a solution. If I did have a solution, I was able to conform to their vision in the best way possible.

This is only one small example of how I mastered an outer pattern. Taking this concept to an extreme stage, I have heard (but not seen) that true spiritual masters exist who can consciously create just about anything through their understanding of the universe's patterns. It is rumored that spiritual masters can manifest things out of thin air. Once a person reaches a high level of enlightenment, he or she can master even the pattern of physical death and rebirth and remain physically immortal, if that is the choice.

But in my life, if I can begin by just understanding that there are patterns in this universe, and if I can slowly take the smallest patterns and learn to understand them and flow with them and ultimately reshape them to fit my vision, then my life as I live it has no limits.

When we fully realize that we have the ability to help shape the universe, we must ask ourselves a question: What is my destiny to contribute to humankind?

Part 3
Tantra and Community

Reaching *13*
Outward

t is such a pleasure to give! I send all the intensity inside my heart straight into him and call on God's love as well. I am mastering his rhythms. I am extending his peak period, so when he orgasms it is so much larger for him. I enjoy having total control of his body and keeping him on that edge of ecstasy for extended periods—to where he is beginning to zone out, go into a trance, just like he does to me.

Today I gave him two orgasms like that, and afterward, it was like he was a changed person, as though new parts of his mind were turning on. He told me he felt as if on drugs but better: there are no side effects. I am making him feel like he makes me feel. It is so nice to be able to give like this. I told him to watch out. I'm beginning to like this now.

I have always marveled at tantra's paradoxical nature. If tantra had a personality, it would be a mischievous imp who softly teases our concepts of right and wrong.

In the past two thousnd years, religion has placed strong restrictions on sexual behavior, as opposed to encouraging sexuality's uninhibited expression. It is important to know that religion can do either. Religion can promote sexual suppression just as easily as it can promote sexual openness.

Whether or not we condone our religion's definition of proper sexual behavior, we can admit its practical side. A thousand years ago sex was a matter of family survival. Making sure your daughter had sex with the right social ally, and no one else, would ensure a pure and unambiguous bloodline. Along with that came a guarantee of keeping the wealth in the family and maintaining political power. A spark of teenage passion might result in an unwanted son who might one day rise to claim ownership of his lawful property. In many cultures it was acceptable for men to have affairs with prostitutes or any other women who were not considered a threat to the family unit. Women, on the other hand, who from one seed can bear a child nine months later, were required to keep a lock and key on their sexuality.

Sexual conduct tells volumes about any given society. Sex has been both decorated and burdened with many customs, rules, and ceremony. We look with eyes biased to our particular culture and have an image of sex that we valiantly uphold. Our cultural image of sex is part of us, just as our personal sexuality is inseparable from our sense of identity. Yet all "norms," sexual and otherwise, are merely one possibility of many that have been chosen by the chains of societies that have come and gone. One thing is for certain: the sexual customs of humanity will change again and again, for the only certainty we face is change.

The Non-Dogma of Sexual Behavior in Tantra

Tantra, like the changing cultural tide of proper sexual behavior, has undergone many permutations. One common debate centers on for whom tantra was meant within the social structure. Tantra has periodically gone underground, away from the prevailing culture. This can be linked to politics. Invading countries usually establish their cultural viewpoints—religion and sexual conduct certainly not the least important—on the original inhabitants of the region. As a result, tantrics lived in communities that were totally separate from their mainstream neighbors—or perhaps they maintained a facade of conformity while practicing in secret, as did the oppressed Jews during the Inquisition. In this role the tantrics of the day would be characterized as persevering and a little rebellious.

Some historians attribute tantra's underground movement to the fact that when political leaders realized tantra's empowerment of the individual, they wanted to use it only for themselves. Leaders feared that tantra would bring power to the masses, who might then upset the social order. Even more cause for alarm is that tantra gives particular power to women. In tantra, men and women share equal status, and equality will always threaten male-dominated societies. In its position to jeopardize, tantra became secretive: an esoteric discipline practiced only by the upper classes, who had the privilege of education and felt more free to break their own rules. As such, tantrics are elitist and wealthy, either upholding great wisdom or feeding their hunger for power.

A third argument comes from the nature of tantra. Any discipline that works with kundalini energies in the body can be dangerous. Kundalini can burn a person from the inside out if it is not properly managed. Tantra is therefore taught orally, from teacher to student on a one-on-one basis with close monitoring. Doing otherwise would be akin to administering heavy medication without a physician's diagnosis. The tantrics in this case are thorough, with spiritual integrity, maintaining tantra's original purpose of enlightenment and oneness with God.

With all this rumor about tantra's secretive past, the ironic discovery is that of its origins. Tantra's roots are from the common people. It evolved from the very early worshiping of the Earth Mother, Gaia, the Creator, the Giver of Life. For proof, look no farther than the earthbound and social nature of tantra. It is not a text-based discipline and does not require reading skills. Tantra is about the pursuit of spiritual liberation in a way that everyone can experience: through earthly pleasure and communion with others. Tantra's true birth was in small villages, within the community, with the simple goal of bringing people together.

Tantra's lineage has come to represent many pieces of the puzzle: enigma, elitism, purity, commonness. Much has been determined by the values of the day. Tantra's fluidity finds a home in many different cultures. Tantra is not revolutionary, for it does not seek to replace what already is. It merges and blends. And it teases.

Even though the picture of tantra has changed, tantra survives on the models of family and community.* Yet although community may be tantra's river, individualism is its sandy bottom that filters impurities. Tantra has always questioned established order. Tantra has always sought to break social taboos by challenging the status quo; however, tantra does not reject social order. Questioning the validity of social structure and custom is tantra's way of adding to society: doing so is the singular cause for the advancement of civilization in all areas. Historical figures such as Einstein, Galileo, Gandhi, and Jesus provide ample example of this. Today we see social advancement in the areas of medical science and technology. Things are getting better because teams of people are questioning what is.

In much of the Western world today, invading enemies generally are not a day-to-day concern for most of us. As we enjoy this time of relative peace, we can turn our minds away from the outside world and look at the oppressions within ourselves. And this is when tantra really shines. Now that most of us live as free men and women—free to choose our religion, sexual conduct, and lifestyle—we have no more excuses to prevent us from finding out what we really want. We can discover our true calling. What is right for me? What is my personal path? Tantra asks that we look within. Tantra does not believe that change will come by altering what is outside of ourselves. It all starts with *me*. Where is the oppression within me? How has my fear of change stopped me from evolving? And how can I do something about it today? Tantra asks that we change what is within us, not that we change a whole society.

But when we change, we unintentionally threaten the established order around us. We disturb the peaceful slumber of those who do not want to awaken—and these sleepers are often those to whom we are closest.

Family, the mirror of society, can be the blessing of true love and fulfillment or the curse of oppression and limitation. Much has to do with how the balance of established order and the need for change—socialization

---

*There are many celibate spiritual paths; tantra is not one of them. Tantra is not a theory; it is a physical, sexual path. The only exception might be the practicing tantric who "retires" to celibacy toward the end of his or her lifetime.

versus individualism—is handled. Like society, families that maintain this delicate balance thrive in harmony and happiness.

Tantra's focus on family and community is something I now cherish. I did not perceive that when I first chose tantra. I thought I wanted tantra because of its newness, its erotic mystery, and because I was such an extreme individualist. Tantra's reliance on others brought up issues within me that I didn't know I had. It made me face my desire to stay separate from others. But if I were only a rebel, choosing this path would have been much easier.

Paradoxically, choosing tantra initially made me feel isolated from the world I had known. My family and childhood friends did not understand what I was doing. Underneath my thin layer of indifference, I wanted to be accepted. I began to see how deep a sense of responsibility I felt to those around me. Responsibility at that point meant doing what others expected of me: in essence, making other people happy. The part of me that cares deeply about what other people think was not the Valerie I projected to the world.

In my case, the worst of all possible consequences happened when I chose a path of tantra. The reactions of my family and friends could not have been worse. At first they thought that I was just going through a phase. As things continued, and their subtle hints did not cause me to change my direction, they started to worry. Had I joined a cult? Against my will? Perhaps I was being brainwashed. And when they discovered that tantra was associated with sex, well, all hell broke loose. You can imagine the fantasies of horror that must have gone through their heads—has their pretty young daughter become entangled in some pagan sex cult that worships the devil? Their reactions caused me considerable grief, because I did not want to upset my relationships. I just wanted to explore who I was. I wanted to become closer to God.

Instead of educating themselves about tantra, or about any discipline of yoga that has similarities to tantra's fundamental principles, my family panicked. They tried to talk to me about the errors of my ways. I listened to their viewpoint, then told them mine. I figured that if I just explained myself logically, they would understand. Wrong! They still thought I must be doing all of this tantra against my will. They then confronted my tantric teachers, but that confused them because my teachers seemed so loving and nice and had very little attachment to whether or not I chose tantra. Then they went to my immediate circle of friends and asked them to keep an eye on me. In other words, they asked my friends to spy. I soon learned who my true friends were. I didn't have many.

All I could feel was betrayal. To have my family blindly reject something that meant so much to me, without even considering that they should respect my ability to make choices, disturbed me deeply. Those whom we love can hurt us the most. I felt as if I had to turn my back on my past.

Western culture does not find it normal to undertake a study with a single teacher. In Eastern religion, a student-guru relationship is a common way of learning. The movie *The Karate Kid* epitomizes the Eastern approach of personalized instruction. But my family had no point of reference for what I was doing. It was not their picture of what was normal. This is the problem with looking at very small pieces of evidence and extrapolating based on a narrow viewpoint. It's the problem that we have when we try to go back and analyze history with our own subjective biases. It is the problem of being so afraid of what is different that we blindly reject it. It is the source of all prejudice and racism. My family believed that in following a path different from theirs I was rejecting their values. But that was really only the surface issue.

When I began to nurse my pain and see beyond the clouds of sadness, I could get a more objective understanding of what their rejection was all about. They had more than justifiable parental worry. Much more.

Certain people in my family did not accept that I was an adult, making my own decisions. They did not consider that I had thoroughly researched tantra, not to mention myriad other spiritual disciplines, and that I was consciously choosing a path that fit *me*

They did not trust that as a woman I could make this type of decision. This showed me what they really thought about women.

They felt insulted that I was making a choice vastly different from theirs. They figured that their way was the right way and the only way. They were, in a word, threatened.

And so, concurrent with the incredible happiness I was feeling through tantra, just as I was truly beginning to understand myself and grow, the relationships around me were crumbling.

I could do one of three things. I could maintain the status quo and choose their way. I could try to change their opinions. Or I could be true to myself and follow my own path.

They didn't understand that some of the good values they'd had taught me were the basis for the decisions I made. I merely questioned the way. I knew in my heart that the way of tantra was right for me. Each spiritual path promotes certain lessons. Tantra emphasizes the enjoyment of life and of community and—ironically—it emphasizes family. How could this possibly be in conflict with the values of my family and friends?

In truth, tantra was never in conflict with their values. They perceived that I was abandoning their ways because I was looking at the world from a different perspective—a perspective that pulled from their values and added my own.

One job I had through college was working as an administrator for an orthodox rabbi. One day he explained to me that even Judaism, one of the oldest religions in the world, holds that Judaism is only one path to God and that all paths to God are valid.

If all paths to God are valid, then what is the right path for me? According to tantra, this question can be answered only by each individual. It cannot be recommended, forced, told, or ordered by anyone else. A spiritual path is a life. Your spiritual path is your life. It is created by you and lived by you.

What is your path?

You already know the answer. It is the simple answer that your heart, your emotions, your body, your spirit knows. You may not accept the answer, but it's there, waiting patiently until you're ready. There's nothing to find. It's already inside you. How can you become something that you already are? Your path must only be accepted and lived.

I chose my own path. But I was left to face the consequences. How did I find my way out of this painful experience? It was to strike a balance. I had to come to know my individualism. Then I had to learn something I was not prepared for.

First the easy part: individualism. Tantra taught me how to focus my mind, body, and emotions so that I could remain centered within my own self without dissolving into the current mood of the family, or blending into the wallpaper, or simply going crazy from the chaos of a life with four parents, four grandparents, five older siblings, a dozen nieces and nephews, a multitude of aunts and uncles, and countless cousins. As I'm sure you know, family have a way of pushing buttons, even if the intention is good. Meditation allowed me to find—and keep—my own power, not to get caught up in all the insanity, and in many cases not to be an instigator of mind games. Simply, it helped me maintain my sense of individuality.

Then came the more unexpected side: an acceptance of my role within the community. Naturally, my first reaction to their rejection was to hold a grudge against them forever. I had no plans to forgive and love my cursed family and friends. Unwillingly, however, I had to admit that it would be better to forgive—not in seven hundred years, but now. Did I mention that tantra is a very fast path? Tantra asks, "Why wait?"

So I had to face the issue. And as I did, the layers peeled away one after the other. I realized that underneath my seething anger was hurt. I was hurt not because of their reaction; I was hurt because I was seeing myself as the helpless child, a victim of this cruel world. In fact, I was seeing myself as others were seeing me. I did not believe that I could really make all my own decisions. I was the weaker sex. I needed their approval to justify my actions because I doubted myself. In fact, we were in perfect agreement.

What a loyal daughter I had become, even in my shallow attempt at rebellion. So I was faced with another choice: I could continue to believe that I was a powerless little girl who was too stupid to make her own decisions or I could change myself. Changing others was not an option (although admittedly I tried!).

At some point in this process I finally understood what my Sunday school teacher kept saying. I really experienced in my heart what it means to turn the other cheek. It means that everything bad that happens outside us is simply a mirror of what is within. Therefore, nothing outside of us can hurt us unless we allow it to. Turning the other cheek means that anything bad someone does to me I can make completely unreal. I can see through that person, that he or she is only my reflection. I can turn inward and see that I have the power to hurt myself or to love myself. Turning the other cheek means to set myself free.

And so I chose the intention to forgive. This was not for the sake of my family. I did it to empower myself. As I forgave, they slowly ceased to control me with a look or a comment or an opinion. I combined this intention to forgive with my practice of tantra. Tantra fueled my thoughts and emotions, to let go of the past and embrace my own power.

Forgiveness and love set us free; anger and pain bind us like prisoners inside our own skin. Forgiveness and love come in small stages, and as the years go by they can become easier and easier. Forgiveness is the only way out of misery, unmet expectations, and hurt within a family and within the world.

And as they say, success is the best remedy when people disapprove. Over the years, my stubborn family has had to admit that my life keeps getting better. I became a much nicer and happier person. I gained more confidence and wisdom. They began to come to me for advice. They were amazed at my level of financial success. I would not let them reject me. I simply stuck around, showed them that their slaps in the face were unreal, and gave them lots of love.

Challenging the
Status Quo

nfinite experiences of pleasure and joy and God. Like drops in the ocean. Like grains of sand. Like people. Who knew there are so many ways to feel pleasure! Each ride he leads me on is totally different. I have no idea how he knows my body so well. I would venture to say that he knows my body better than even I do. Some orgasms are quite deep, and I feel them not by the contractions of my yoni; I feel them inside of my blood. I feel my body lie motionless, unbreathing, and my heart is beating and I can almost hear the blood; all I hear and feel is my heart and my blood. This is the internal orgasm. It rises, the pulsing, rising and rising, like a wave of light running loose inside me, going deeper and higher . . . and it ends in silence. It ends when I take a breath.

If ever there is an area where tantra adds to society, it's within the realm of relationships. The forms of relationships in tantra have been both similar to and different from conventional relationships. Much has depended on the culture around which tantra was implemented.

India, the birthplace of tantra, is a sexually conservative culture, much more so than is America. The sexual tantric path is the shame of modern India, and in ancient India it was even worse. As in many patriarchal societies, women were considered property and it was preferable to bear sons. This was partly a financial issue: the bride's parents had to pay a dowry to the husband's family for each daughter who married. This meant that a family with all girls could lose its wealth. On the other hand, each son had the potential to bring his family wealth when he married. Because of this system, sex had to be controlled.

From its inception tantra has always been pushing boundaries.

Tantric Ashrams and Communities

One positive influence of India's culture on tantra is the ashram model. An ashram, like a church, a synagogue and a mosque, is a place of spiritual worship. Usually it is inhabited by a spiritual teacher who has made his or her spiritual path the one and only purpose in life. This teacher will accept students who come to him seeking the same spiritual path. A student may live with the teacher for any amount of time—three months or thirty years—depending on the individual. This program of total immersion allows a one-on-one spiritual training geared specifically to each student.

Another benefit of the ashram is the focus on the greater good as opposed to that of the individual. The ashram is designed to deprogram our years of self-absorption, or the ego's concentration from birth on "me." The ashram cares about the collective good. In order to let go of the self completely, the student renounces all personal ambitions, possessions, and attachments with an extreme sense of humility that says, "I am nothing, and the collective is everything." This form of humility is encouraged and built into the ashram model so that the student can release the self from patterns of self-absorbtion and once again find a balance. Any spiritual relationship requires a deep level of intimacy and trust, and in tantra we are using all parts of ourselves in intimacy: our minds, our hearts, and our bodies.

Tantric ashrams still exist in certain parts of India. Sadly, some have degenerated to places of prostitution. Do not mistake this devolution as tantra. As in most parts of the world today, sexuality in India has a dual face. True tantric ashrams are not about easy or kinky sex. The original purpose of a tantric ashram is to be a place where a student can come and learn about love in a structured, safe environment. It is similar in style to a monastery. My partner once told me a story about his teacher, Sunyata Saraswati. Sunyata was an American man who, many years ago, went to India to learn about tantra. India is critical of outsiders coming over to learn tantra, because Westerners tend to be fascinated by sex. Impressed with Sunyata's sincerity, however, they allowed him to come in and learn. When he entered the ashram, he saw many young and beautiful women whose acquaintance he would love to make. Imagine learning all about God in such an environment! Could a man envision anything more heavenly? But his teacher was wise, and wanted him to see beyond his own visual desires. The teacher led him to an old, wrinkled woman whose beauty had faded many years before. There was nothing Sunyata found arousing about this woman. But when they practiced tantra, she did things to him that he will remember for the rest of his life.

Because my study with my tantric teacher has been so successful, it is my hope that one day we will have successful tantric ashrams in the West that are condoned by society. These would be schools similar to the ashram model of the East, in which a student enters for a certain length of time to study the art of tantra. This ashram model would uphold the guru-student relationship that seems to work so well, because a spiritual path is very personal. It would ensure the integrity of tantra by not allowing any of the misuse of the practice. A Western tantric ashram would need to be modernized. We cannot drop our work, education, and social lives and do nothing but have tantric sex for months or years on end. The model could be something like a college extension course, or like a fully employed graduate program in which a student comes to study the art of tantra in the evenings or on weekends for several years.

In our society, where ashrams are not the norm, we find the *tantric community*. This is a gathering of families who practice tantra, but still go about their normal everyday lives. Most tantric communities remain quite private because of the controversial nature of tantra. But they are out there, if you look closely. In tantric communities, tantra is generally practiced between married couples or adult partners. In some communities all partners get together once a month for a spiritual celebration—this is where the famous *chakra puja* comes into play. (A discussion of this sex ritual is in chapter 15.)

In most countries there are both private teachers and organizations that promote tantra. Most tantric teachers and organizations offer workshops that vary both in level of experience, from beginners to advanced, and in duration, from one to ten days. Most also offer private consultations. Some offer tantric teacher training. Workshops are probably the easiest way to get an introduction to tantra. Introductory courses usually take place on a weekend. The investment, which ranges from $200 to $600, is well worth it. A workshop held by reputable teachers is a very safe environment in which to learn tantra (for a list of recommended teachers, see the appendix). But any workshop will take you only to the starting line, because tantric study requires diligent, repetitive tantric lovemaking.

Relationship Forms

Just as it is in our personal lives, the fundamental core from which social growth is possible is safety. There is great fear to be perceived in relationships—fear of hurting another emotionally, fear of being hurt. Today the threat of AIDS adds a physical danger. There will be no widespread sexual liberation until there is a cure for AIDS. Like the wise turtle, we will not come out of our shells if we do not perceive absolute safety in the world around us. We're smart. We won't allow ourselves to expand our minds and our boundaries unless we first create a context of total emotional safety. Tantra can supply a context of safety, and this all centers on a core that we keep coming back to: an intention of love.

Everything around us indicates that the human race is advancing at exponential rates. In the fields of medicine, technology, archaeology, and science we are aggregating as a global consciousness. Humankind will look back at us in a hundred years and call this time a Golden Age. (Either that, or they will say we were really backward but on the right track!) Within our relationships, it is no different. We itch to break out of the confines of established rules and grow, expand, advance. Half of all marriages end in divorce; there must be something we are missing. We crave the exploration of undiscovered places in our hearts. We wish to examine the very definition of *relationship,* the ways in which we love. We wish to question our boundaries. We wish to ask, "What if?"

Relationship Models

Today, monogamy is the predominant acceptable form of a relationship. One benefit of monogamy is clear: it can offer a context of extreme closeness and deep trust. Loving one person totally is the easiest place from which to begin to open our hearts.

Polygamy (one husband with multiple wives) has been adopted by many cultures in various parts of the world, including China, India, some Arab nations, Japan, and ancient Rome and Greece. Most women today consider polygamy to be patriarchal because, in their perception, it does not put women on an equal level. Contemporary women may assume that one whole woman should get one whole man. Why should she have to share?

There is definitely much evidence in history of polygamy going hand in hand with chauvinism and a patriarchal model. But why do we assume that all women in polygamous cultures in the past would have preferred monogamy? An incorrect assumption made in modern analysis is that polygamous relationships were negative and unfulfilling for women. We look at the past with our twenty-first-century goggles and assume that all women hated this arrangement. And yet—lacking a time machine—we can never really know what they felt about the experience.

What we do know is that we can expect polygamy, like all cultural phenomena, to manifest itself very differently under varied contexts of race, culture, region, time period, and religion. It is interesting to speculate how polygamy would be accepted today, for instance, when we are finally beginning to break out of the patriarchal model. In today's world, polygamy would be the mutual decision of the man and the woman, both of whom are capable of financially supporting themselves.

Polyandry is one wife with many husbands—a more female-centric model that has virtually no popularity. It may be that polyandry hasn't been popular because, given the survival needs of agrarian-based cultures, it has simply been more practical for a man to have more wives rather than the reverse. It may follow that as we continue the current trend of new social terms set forth by industrialization—including shared labor division between men and women in both the public and private sectors—that it is more practical to explore a polyandrous model.*

Together Forever by Charles P. Brown (Eternal Flame Foundation, 1990) received much media attention as a result of this threesome "marriage" with one woman and two men.

Polyamory, a partnership among multiple men and women, is the name for the mature form of the experimentalism that gained popularity through the 1960s.* In this scenario, each man and woman might have one main spouse or partner, but also interact intimately with others within the community. This is not the same as the "swinging" movement where two married couples would swap partners for the night. Polyamory means being in a closed community, and the intimacy reaches far beyond a sexual fling for the night. Polyamory implies commitment on multiple levels between partners. The whole idea is to create a supportive, loving, and fulfilling community—those old-fashioned, small-town principles that sometimes seem to be forgotten in today's world.

If we think we can be in love only once, or with just one person, we are underestimating our hearts. Love is not a finite mechanism. Our ability to love others is vaster than we can imagine. We have an infinite capacity for love. Take the example of a mother of six. She does not love each child less, as if she must divide the amount of love within her heart by six. She takes care of each one, loving each child separately with all the space in her heart. Consider your personal network of friends and family. Have you ever told yourself, "I now have too many friends. I have no more space in my heart for another person." Sure, you may not have time for more friends. You may not have more room in your car for carrying more people to a baseball game. But those are the facts of the physical universe, and our hearts are not bound by that physical universe.

Our hearts are capable of infinite loving. Within tantra, the form of the relationship doesn't matter in the least. Tantra can fit into many different types of relationships—all you really need is two people. But to human beings, form matters very much, and that's why tantra probes at the issue. It forces us to look outside our little minds and look at life in a different context. By acknowledging other ways of loving, we can consciously ask ourselves, "What is right for me?" Established norms are just that —established norms. They should be a place from which we make our own decisions about the relationship models that will make us happy. Ultimately, it is not our

---

Polyamory: The New Love Without Limits by Deborah Anapol (Intinet Resource Center, 1997). Dr. Anapol has been a vocal advocate for the polyamory movement in the western United States.

parents, not our country, not even our church that defines what is right for us—we decide for ourselves.

We make the world a better place when we live according to our inner voices. Despite whether others may acknowledge this, when we are happy we are able to respond to those around us in a better, more positive way.

Constitutionally, the United States is built around the core of religious tolerance. By no means have we built a perfect political model—political perfection is an oxymoron. But religious tolerance does work, as do its corollaries: acceptance of ethnic diversity and freedom of speech. It is time for relationship tolerance. It is time that we move beyond our Victorian prudishness and, by acknowledging and learning from the diversity of other cultures, create stronger and better models of relationships. If I choose monogamy from a standpoint of freedom, by first questioning and looking and knowing that this way is not the only way, my monogamous life will be so much stronger, and I will not fall into that "ball-and-chain" trap. Perhaps that's why so many marriages fail today—it's not a conscious choice, it's just something you do. This is not to say that polylove is better than monogamy. But the exclusion of either is wrong. Fortunately, tantra has no bias. Monogamy will work perfectly well in a tantric lifestyle. What tantra does assert is: Know thyself; do not fear thy hidden desires.

Sexual Preference

My discovery of tantra challenged my own personal views of myself as a heterosexual, monogamous woman. I found this quite disconcerting. The lifestyle of my tantric teachers was enough to get me questioning. I struggled. Why was I afraid to examine my own personal views about relationships? After all, anything of value and truth must be able to withstand intense scrutiny and questioning. Otherwise it's but a flimsy shell that I couldn't rely on anyway, and I was better off knowing that from the start.

I discovered a new part of myself: my physical attraction to women in addition to men. The thought frightened me. I feared that even considering something like that might turn me into a lesbian. Here I was, a seemingly open-minded, confident woman, afraid of my own sexuality. Or perhaps I was more afraid of what others would think. Once I let these suppressed feelings about women rise to the surface without judgment, I realized that it was my denial, not my newly discovered feelings, that had been causing me pain. When we fear that a thought or feeling will hurt us, we tend to suppress that thought because we assume that it will cause us to become something we do not want to be. But we are always in control. The only time we are not in control is when we are suppressing our feelings. Just because I feel something does not mean I need to act upon it or abandon my control over my choices. My feelings merely showed me, once again, that love could not be contained within my narrow framework of what love should look like. As I acknowledged my attraction to women, I realized that I was not a lesbian, nor was I less attracted to men. I had simply become conscious of yet another part of myself and my sexuality. I retained the choice of whether I wished to explore this part or not.

This was simply my experience. Most women delving into tantra will not have identical issues to the ones I found on my path. If tendencies are not inside us to begin with, tantra will not create them. It is not possible for tantra to cause our innate sexual preferences to change.

Jealousy

One of the greatest challenges in love of any kind is jealousy. There is nothing easy about overcoming big, ugly jealousy. When we think we're over it, it comes up again. But contrary to popular opinion, jealousy is not a function of love. Jealousy is a negative lower emotion originating from the feeling of loss. Jealousy has nothing to do with love.

Some of us find it perfectly normal that our parents love us and our siblings and that their loving our siblings does not preclude loving us. If we feel any loss, we at least understand it, and realize that soon enough we will get our time with Mom or Dad. But logic goes out the window when we have romantic love or—to put it bluntly—when we have sex with someone. Why do sexual relationships incite jealousy? It always seems to come back to sex. Sexuality is so linked with our sense of identity that those with whom we share our sexuality also become tightly linked with our sense of identity. Our partners become an emotional extension of us.

Just as we hold tightly to our sense of identity, finding it difficult to change our core personality, so do we grasp our sexual partners as though they are our possessions. Afraid to surrender who we think we are, we become afraid to surrender our possessions.

To add even more complication, we can thank our Neanderthal ancestors for genetically passing down our blind possessiveness. It's a matter of survival. We want our genes only to perpetuate. But possessiveness and jealousy have nothing to do with love. Love is infinite. Love gives. I chose a spiritual path because I could feel the shackles around my heart. Initial lessons dealt with my own problems and issues. I had to know myself. Then I had to love myself. Over time, as I let go of possession of my identity, and especially my identity as a sexual woman, the shackles disappeared. But freeing myself was only the first step. The next step was to set free the people I love—in particular, to set free my lover, the man I think of as an extension of myself. Could I possibly set him free? Could I give up that much control? What is the meaning of unconditional love? What does an open heart mean? Can I be so much at one with my mate that I can enjoy him physically, intimately loving another person, because all I care about is his happiness? The very thought of setting my lover free got my heart racing with the raging fire of jealousy. How hypocritical I was! *Here I am, a woman who practices tantric lovemaking with a tantric teacher who is a married man.* How could I expect my boyfriend not to be jealous when I myself was so possessive?

Thus, I decided to confront this demon that had hold of me. And like any surface emotion, jealousy melted when I saw what was lying underneath: *I am not worthy of being loved.* A remnant of the divorce between my parents? Does it really matter where the thought came from? And beneath even this lay the most painful belief I have ever faced, and that is the belief that I am separate from others, and that I am somehow cut off from God's love.

Then I discovered the group-sex rituals of tantra.

Tantric
Sex Rituals

n my dreams I am the Goddess tonight. I am the experienced one who is served as an offering to the group. They lay me down on the earth, they place offerings of food and wine on me, they feed off my body, sucking my breasts, groping my hips, licking my fingers and toes and arms and legs. I am the initiator of all who seek oneness. I take into me the young men who are this night virgins, whose swollen virility finds home in my folds. I hold them in a womblike embrace, and I let them howl and whimper and cry for the mother they seek, the Goddess they adore.

I am the trusting sister the young girls desire. Seeking to know themselves, they approach me, timid. I answer with softness, teaching them to respect themselves and treat each other as goddesses always, teaching through touch, through a soft tongue that reaches tenderly into their small mouths and opens them, opens them to the Moon's call. My hands are the guide and my tongue reassures their questions and they trust, trust. They trust my tongue, which turns their desire into a throb and into a frenzy, and when they surrender to the climax it is themselves, their true selves, their true hearts that they surrender to. In this dream I am the deliverer of remembrance.

Tantra is not the inventor of sex ritual; there is evidence of sex ritual in many societies. But because the predominant religions for the past two thousand years forbade ritual, especially Judeo-Christian culture, we don't hear about it much in school. Western history books omit the topic entirely.

Yet some lingering customs come directly from sex rituals. Valentine's Day is the descendant of the Lupercalian festivals during the first century B.C. in ancient Rome. These festivals, which took place in February in honor of a goddess of love, Juno Februata, were held in purification to the New Year and to honor the spirit of love. These festivals consisted of sex rituals in which all participants' names were written on paper and sexual partners for the evening were randomly selected. This custom evolved into the modern-day tradition of sending Valentine's Day cards.* (This celebration eventually became Christianized in memory of Saint Valentine, who was associated with the union of lovers under conditions of duress.)

There is the famous Maypole dance in which girls and boys coming of age would dance around this phallic symbol and then spend the night together in the woods, celebrating their own symbols. (Some women's groups celebrate the May*hole* dance, for reasons we can infer.)

Then there are festivals, such as the famous European Carnival Festival, during which nothing is forbidden on that day. India has a similar Holi, the festival celebrating plant life that forbids very little.†

The purpose of sex rites varies, from honoring the divine to ensuring fruitful crops. The Dionysian Mysteries in ancient Greece are where we get the actual term *orgy*. In these rituals it was thought that sexual worship would bring about human fertility. These rituals began as a grassroots effort, and later the festival came under the control of the state, being held twice annually as an official celebration. Andre Van Lysebeth, in *Tantra: The Cult of the Feminine*, says of the tantric sex rituals known as *chakra puja:* "they are an extension of the ancient fertility rites when collective intercourse was performed in the fields and was thought to promote fertility, not only of human beings, but of animals and crops as well."‡

*Sarah Dening, *The Mythology of Sex* (UK: Macmillan, 1996): 82.
†Andre Van Lysebeth, *Tantra: The Cult of the Feminine*, 281.
‡Ibid., 278.

Through these ancient rites, we see how sex becomes synonymous with abundance: abundance of food (crops), abundance of children (fertility), abundance of comfort (good weather). Is this surprising? Sex, after all, is the only means of continuing the human race.

Sex is associated with the abundance of wealth. Whenever a society experiences great prosperity, people express more liberal views of sexuality. This is true with the Golden Ages of the Greeks and Romans, the prosperous Etruscans, and the wealthy Victorians. We even see this in the Bible, when powerful kings such as Solomon had hundreds of wives. In our contemporary time we continue to witness the interrelationship between sex and wealth. During prosperous ecomonic times we see signs of sexual liberation, such as the seductive clothing of women in the late 1920s. In the early 1960s and early 1970s, for example, when our economy was at a high, the hippie and disco movements led us in a "sexual revolution." Inversely, sexual tensions in society can affect economies. AIDS—the ultimate inhibitor of sex—became a worldwide epidemic in the late 1980s. In 1989 a financial recession swept the nation. The unconscious archetype continues its uncanny pattern.

As this book is going into publication we have not yet found a cure for AIDS, and we still feel too afraid to open our sexuality. Once we find both a cure and a vaccine against this deadly virus, there will be a strong resurgence of sexual liberalism.

In my experience group sex ritual is the ultimate expression of tantra's immersion in community. But not all tantrics practice group sex ritual. It is highly misunderstood, both in its purpose and in its details. In fact tantric sex ritual is the only way that I have been able to heal my personal sense of jealousy, underneath which lay the desperate feeling that I was separate from God.

That last fact deserves repeating: Tantric sex ritual helped me heal my jealousy issue. You cannot imagine how surprising I found this.

There are two main tantric sex rituals, both of which are still practiced in parts of India and China. These are the *maithuna* (see chapter 5) and the *chakra puja*. In the flavor of true ritual, mystery and secrecy surround them. *Chakra puja* can be translated as "worship practiced in a circle." Both rituals share the purpose of transformation of consciousness and, ultimately, enlightenment. The goal is to experience the divinity, the light of God, within our partners.

Both rituals involve the Five Steps, also called the Five Makaras. The Five Makaras are each aspect of Indian culture that are strictly forbidden. Again we see how tantra questions the established dogma of social order. These "steps" are: wine, meat, fish, grains (traditionally aphrodisiac grains), and ritual lovemaking. This is where the similarities of maithuna and chakra puja end, however.

The maithuna, as we know, celebrates the relationship with our partners; think of the chakra puja of as an affirmation of our personal relationship with God.

The chakra puja gets a bad rap when we judge it by today's ethical standards. We're all deeply conditioned to know what's right and what's wrong, especially when it comes to sex. Good girls and boys do only certain "normal" things, and anything outside that realm of normalcy we must consider kinky or dirty, if for no reason other than to maintain our semblance of dignity.

But the purpose of this ritual is highly spiritual. The chakra puja, being quite different from the maithuna in practice, still upholds the basic purpose of enlightenment and oneness. The chakra puja traditionally corresponds with the cycle of the Moon. It is held monthly, usually during the full moon. The full moon represents the time at which we surrender. Women shed their menses, and as farmers know, no seeds are planted in the earth. It is a time to let go.

The puja is held in a group setting, usually with eight couples. In this ceremony the man is not to ejaculate. The chakra puja especially honors the female, or rather the female qualities within us, or the principle of *shakti*.*
This ritual takes place in the evening, in a place of privacy. An equal number of men and women sit in a circle. One couple consists of the guru and his shakti. Here is where things change. Although every woman came with her

---

Shakti is the Sanskrit term for the female principle, and *Shiva* is the corresponding male principle. Shakti and Shiva can also represent a goddess and god, respectively. In tantra we worship our partners as containing the divinity of Shakti or of Shiva.

spouse or partner, it is now time to change mates. Either randomly or by the guidance of the guru, the men and women separate and link up with another partner. This new couple will be ritualistically wedded for the night, and every person in the group is in accord with this. It is furthermore agreed that the new joining couple will have no relations or affairs outside of this ritual, for that would be forbidden by tantric standards.

This "marriage" is one of metaphor only; obviously the participants do not really get married. The reason for this ritualistic marriage is in some ways contrary to the maithuna, which is an affirmation of the relationship we have. At the chakra puja it is the goal to transcend the normal concept of what we define as a romantic relationship. A romantic relationship can be exclusionary and possessive. Romantic love also carries expectations of and judgments about our partners. Expectation and judgment thwart unconditional love.

Thus united with new partners who are virtualy strangers, the negative emotional aspects of a committed relationship are temporarily put aside. We can now meditate on the true, almost impersonal divinity of every living thing.

Conversely, being in love with a stranger for one night means that we have to let go of the idea that our partners or spouses are the only people worthy of our care, effort, and unconditional love. It may be easy for me to see the divinity in my husband, for he is the father of my children, my provider and caretaker. I am now being asked to enter into a divine meditation with a total stranger, with whom I have no background, who could be a total jerk for all I know! But the goal is to go beyond all these self-centered expectations about love. The purpose of chakra puja is to let ourselves experience unconditional love, for no other purpose than the love itself in this moment.

The chakra puja involves the five makaras of wine, meat, fish, grain, and sexual union. The guru, as host for the evening, guides the ceremony as a strict regimen. His partner is a beautiful and young woman who lies in the center of the circle, symbolizing the divine female. The couples together share the five makaras in a ritual meal, partake in chanting and prayer, and then consummate their "marriage" through very controlled intercourse. As in the maithuna, there is hardly any movement. All couples remain conscious of the divinity of their partners and focus on the energy flowing between them. The guru guides the couples into various positions and breathing techniques. This group meditation ends with the women achieving orgasm and the men retaining the energy of their ejaculation, pulling it inward and upward in order to use it to transcend their own consciousness.

When I experienced my first chakra puja, the event marked an even deeper strengthening of my spiritual connection to others. At this point in my life I was feeling strong enough to merge this separation between my spiritual life and my romantic relationships. I wanted more integration. Just as I was now bringing romance and passion into my relationship with my tantric partner, I also wanted to bring tantra into my romantic relationships. I wanted to experience what it feels to be totally in love with someone and totally spiritually connected at the same time.

My relationship with my tantric partner has also become very strong. He had become my best friend, my confidant, and my support system. Perhaps I wanted more from him than just a tantric relationship. Perhaps I wanted something more sustaining. It began to feel as though I was *dating* him, as though he was my boyfriend. Under the circumstances, this direction simply was not the purpose of our relationship. I accepted this fact, but the conflict remained. I felt as if I were dating two people at once: my boyfriend and my tantric partner.

This desire within me led me to invite my then boyfriend to a tantric workshop. He was very open-minded about it. I had accomplished step one: a boyfriend who was genuinely interested in practicing tantra!

I was nervous about the workshop. Not every tantric workshop ends in a puja, but this one—as the materials disclosed—would. I didn't particularly want to share my boyfriend with a roomful of other women or, for that matter, to be drooled on by strange men. Until now most of my experience consisted of monogamous tantra with my one and only tantric partner.

My boyfriend and I discussed the imminent chakra puja in great detail. We both confessed our fear, anxiety, excitement—the gamut of emotions that sex tends to bring up. We agreed that during the puja we would remain together as a couple, for we did not want to be hooked up with strangers. We vowed that the purpose of our participation in this workshop would be to learn tantra together and strengthen our relationship. Still, I was not satisfied with just that: I had horrific images of my boyfriend being swarmed by a dozen young, beautiful tantrikas and leaving me in the corner somewhere collecting dust. My boyfriend wanted to do everything he could to alleviate my fear, so the second agreement we made was that I could choose what we would and would not do—in other words, he would follow my lead. (In the tradition of tantra, the woman's feelings are almost always put first.) Third, we vowed that either of us could veto what the other was doing simply by saying so. This rhetoric lasted hours until we finally arrived at our destination, doing much to make us feel close.

Communication is still the best way to achieve oneness. Plus, as any woman will attest, it's the greatest aphrodisiac!

The workshop center, nestled high in the mountains, was built of wood with vaulted ceilings that captured the sun's warmth. We were somewhat taken aback by the crowd, about forty people; they were of all ages, all backgrounds, and, against the backdrop of my imaginative mind, seemed surprisingly normal. There were some basic rules of this three-day tantric workshop. First, clothing was optional. Second, they encouraged that lovemaking be performed only in public, not in privacy. You can imagine the diffidence along with anticipation that this skewing of "normal behavior" brought about.

The instructors, a man and a woman, had us break into smaller groups of eight, with equal numbers of males and females. We called our own group Isis. We proceeded to spend Friday and Saturday becoming very close. There is something that nudity does to melt the walls of emotional distance. It creates a natural context to share more of ourselves in a brief amount of time. In Isis we did nearly everything together. We practiced workshop exercises together, such as breathing and visualization. We ate together. We bathed in hot tubs together. We basked in the sun together. Some of us even slept in the same room together. Yet there was no lovemaking. We were just people getting to know each other, learning some fundamental things about tantra. We were of very different backgrounds. Still, we became very close, letting our emotional inhibitions fall away so that more of our hearts could shine through.

The anticipated chakra puja came on Saturday evening. By this time I had no idea where my paranoid, fearful mind had gone, but I was not about to go looking for it. I was entirely at peace. I felt closer to my boyfriend than

I ever had, although we had not made love and had spent hardly any time alone. Neither of us had used our right to veto, and I had not imposed my will on him even once, although it was somehow comforting to know that I had that right.

On Saturday before sunset, the men and women prepared for the celebration separately. We had two requirements: to come dressed in something that made us feel sensual and to bring one food offering. The women gathered together and we helped each other bathe, do our hair, and dress. The communal bonding among women is so important, for it makes us realize that we are not each other's enemies. There is a special connection among women that is found nowhere else. In helping to prepare each other, we honored ourselves, we honored the sacred Shakti. Seductive, perfumed, and warmed from the soft pampering, just before sunset the women entered the room in which our men awaited us with great anticipation.

We sat in a circle, holding hands, and said a prayer for healing and transformation of consciousness. A large pit of sand piled with rocks lay in the center of the circle.* The gurus (instructors) asked us to go, one by one, into the center of the circle and pick up a rock. This was the symbol of whatever heavy baggage, resistance, or walls we wished to let go of, or break down tonight and forever. As we went around the circle, we dropped our rocks into the sandpit and announced what we consciously chose to get rid of.

I had no idea what I wanted to let go of; I had too many options. It wasn't until I stood over the sand that I heard a voice from within a tiny spot in my heart.

I will let go of my fear of love.

And with the utterance of those words a heavy weight seemed to lift from my chest. For despite years of tantric practice, there was a part of me that had always held back. With this rock I tossed out my heavy burden of fear and saw that the fear was not so large, not so oppressive—it was hardly larger than a lump of coal. I guess this is how all fear is—it feels enormously heavy until we bring it into the light and examine it.

When each participant had spoken, the gurus lit the container in which

---

*Sand is symbolic of protection.

the rocks were held and a small bonfire erupted, the flames seeming to lick the rocks, cleansing the debris of the group.

Music began, and a drummer beat his shaman's drum, uniting the music's rhythm to the rhythm of the group. The room smelled of rich sandalwood and fire. Food and juice were passed around the circle. My taste buds seemed to explode with each delicious morsel. We were hardly moving, sitting in this circle, focusing on the pure experience of the moment, eating a small offering from each bowl that was passed. I felt my heart softening, felt a profound connection to this group. Everyone seemed unusually beautiful, and pure, and perfect to me.

Our palates satiated, it was now time for the circle ritual. The women stood outside the circle while the men remained sitting, now facing us. Each woman faced one man. The music intensified. Honoring each man in turn, the women slowly danced and moved around the circle, honoring the men through the love in our eyes, through the sensuous motion of our bodies, through our acknowledgment of their divinity. We became the incarnation of feminine divinity: the mother, the daughter, the sister, the seductress. Mother Earth's soothing energy rose through our feet, up our thighs, through our sex, into our spines, and out our hearts. We brought each man into the aura of our hearts without touching, without words. With each inhale we brought in the divine mother and with each exhale we touched their hearts more deeply.

The men then danced for the women, and the spiritual elation we were enjoying as a group flowed into joy, for who will not delight in seeing grown men dancing for women? They honored us now, the divine substance within us, through gaze and movement, through the soft valiance that is uniquely special to men. Their dancing was of desire, the desire of wanting to understand and contain all of the unpredictability and sensitivity of a woman, to hold a gentle space for her to feel completely safe to let go and trust. They were the teacher and guide, pioneer of freedom, keeper of integrity, provider. They were the father, the brother, the son. Fueled with the light of father God that danced up their spines and out through their hearts and into us, they became the symbol of creation and life. Loving respect poured from their eyes and into our hearts.

Through this dance we let our judgments and walls dissolve, releasing all thought except consciousness of the God in all of us, the God that courses through every cell in our bodies, the God that is the substance of our souls, the God that is everywhere and all.

Then we broke into our smaller families, and I was reunited with my group, Isis. Now was time for the ritual massage. The gurus told us that we could do this with just our partners or with an anonymous partner for the evening, in the tradition of chakra puja. Without speaking, my boyfriend and I knew our choice. So did the whole of Isis, as though we were now eight people with one mind. We would perform the ritual together, as a unit. My heart exploded with love and peace.

With massage oil that smelled of sensuous musk, we anointed our family, two at a time, while one man and one woman lay on the floor. Three people massaged one person, then switched. We were instructed to channel the excitement of this exercise into our hearts by focusing on the divinity of the man and woman in front of us. At this point it was not difficult to concentrate, even with the sexual energy flowing through us. Perhaps it was easy, because when I looked at the faces of my group, all I could see was a joyous mindfulness. We were moved, experiencing a place within our hearts that we could not normally reach. As I massaged, I could see nothing but the perfection of each woman and man of Isis. There was depth to each one of them. There were vulnerability, strength, and potential. Why had I not seen this so clearly before? Why did I spend my time judging, or feeling threatened, or believing I was different or separate from my boyfriend, my friends, my brothers and sisters, my family?

My boyfriend and I were the last of Isis to be ritually massaged. The feeling of six pairs of hands lovingly stroking my body was beyond anything I had known. The pleasure was profound—as though every inch of my body could reach orgasm by their touch. For the first time in my life in any kind of group setting, I let go. I let myself receive. I put up no barriers. Streams of tears poured down my face: they were of both joy and relief and sadness for all the times that I could not let myself shine through. Why had I waited so long? Why had I held on to my fear so tightly?

The beautiful women of Isis, my sisters, lovingly massaged my boyfriend. I didn't know where my jealousy and possessiveness had gone. I couldn't find them. It was as though my whole mind had shifted to another context of thinking, where such emotions did not make any sense. All I could see and feel and desire were his total happiness and their total happiness. I let go. I set him free.

The sensuality lasted for several hours after the massage. I channeled all my passion and spiritual elation into my boyfriend. When I looked into his eyes as we made love, I felt that I could see God. We could feel the bliss in the room, like currents of electricity sweeping through the air. Now it would have been easy for the passion to get out of control. But the gurus, wise to understand that the source of the real excitement was God, continued to channel our passion, gently reminding us to lift all the passion upward into our hearts, and kept our minds focused on God. And this, it must be known, was the source of infinite pleasure. God is what made tantra infinitely more pleasurable than normal sex, or any type of orgy, for that matter. The chakra puja was everything I had practiced in a smaller setting, but with the added energy of this group. We were celebrating the infinite current of joy that is God together.

The chakra puja is the only group ritual activity within tantra. Its intention is to unite people with the core purpose of becoming more aware of God. Any tantric sex ritual that does not leave you feeling this way is not tantra. There are many false paths that will use the guise of tantra as an excuse to have group sex. I wouldn't say there is anything wrong with group sex if all involved are consenting adults. But don't mistake those events for tantra.

The chakra puja changed a lifelong perception I had about love. It changed not only my mental belief, but also my emotional experience from a context that love must be limited and possessed, to a true context of love's eternal expansion. It's the only thing that helped me go beyond jealousy. The puja erodes the source of jealousy, which is that we are separate from the men and women around us.

That night I saw the God in my partner, and God can always be trusted. Because I saw only his divinity, there was nothing for me to fight or guard against. Through the perception of our divinity, nothing can be taken away from us because we already have everything. I'm not saying that in a flash I was cured of jealousy and a sense of separation forever. But it did give me the place from which to start. The key is to establish repetition, so that these moments of oneness come more and more often. Over many years, true change occurs.

People learn many different lessons from the chakra puja. But all lessons have one thing in common: all have to do with how we feel within the community. The next morning, when we were again assembled in a circle, we went around the group and shared our experiences. One man said it transformed his relationship with other men because instead of being combative and competitive, he experienced the support of the men during the most intimate of all possible occasions. A woman, who had been extremely self-conscious about her weight, shared that it was the first time she felt comfortable with her body. Another man, who was seen as an aloof loner, admitted that he was finally beginning to like people. The puja teaches about love and oneness. As a group, we learned to love ourselves more, others more, and God more.

Part 4
Path of God

Final 16
Resistance

saw a thousand-petal lotus residing in my heart. His licks gently stroked each individual petal. I called upon God to be with me, and indeed I felt him. He is always there when I ask for him, sometimes when I feel him during such intensity I want to cry, it fulfills me so. The combination of total physical pleasure with total spiritual pleasure— what else is there worth living for? How much better does it get?

Bodies pulsating in sweat, rich with the scent of arousal, an eternal moment away from orgasm. Unaware of the space defining this room, or the time of day, or my name. I have reached an edge of forever just before orgasm and gone beyond it—into what feels like a different dimension, a saturated emptiness, the pregnant womb of origin.

I have become pleasure.

And now, yes, finally, my orgasm.

But no! Pain is all I feel. An intensity, yes, but not the pleasure I had awaited. Never before, never before. Why is tantra hurting me? Could it be that my anchor of safety and happiness is capable of inflicting pain?

This experience, which happened in the eighth year of my commitment to tantra, shined a light upon my wall of resolution. There was a chink in my willful armor. Somewhere inside, I doubted my decisions.

Every tantric experience until now—every small step along the path—had brightened my world with unexpected happiness, always exceeding my expectations. Tantra is my path of freedom. Limited by nothing, I grow upward, into the truth of who I am. Tantra is my personal inner sanctuary of safety, aliveness, and love.

But what was I to make of this painful orgasm?

As I silenced my fear and once again found my center of clarity, I began to doubt my moment of doubt.

When a lemon is empirically tested, its flavor is not bitter as we experience it. Its fruit is incredibly sweet, more so than the ripest strawberry dipped in chocolate and pure cane sugar. However, the lemon's sweet juices are beyond the range of our taste buds, and its acid confuses our senses—we likely spit its bitter aftertaste from our puckered lips.

Once again I was facing the limitations of my physical spectrum.

At the time of my overwhelming orgasm, my partner's tongue was dancing on my yoni light as a feather. There was absolutely no pain before the orgasm. In fact, the pleasure was encompassing me like the sun on a hot summer day. The only difference was in the duration of the build. I had remained on that verge just before orgasm for an unusually long time—nearly three hours.

Before the orgasm I was riding waves of immense delight. During the orgasm, those waves became enormous. I had never swum such huge currents. The orgasm was bigger than I. The pleasure was more than my body was trained to contain at one time.

The orgasm was not a source of pain, but instead a gift showing me a glimpse of ecstasy patiently awaiting my embrace. It was I who must be willing to go beyond my range of experience. To see the next horizon, even before my eyes were adjusted to the light, meant that I was growing.

That, and I should know what to expect the next time I enjoy three hours of tantric foreplay.

Children have no predefined range of what they will let themselves feel: emotionally, physically, and even spiritually. We would be wise to learn from children. As adults it becomes easy to slowly but steadily stop learning and growing. It becomes easy to let our comfort zones stay the same or, even worse, deteriorate until we are as rigid as grumpy, old people waiting for death.

Our perceptions and experiences of spirituality are similarly at risk of stagnation. The *spiritual comfort zone* is the sum total of everything we think about God. What we experience of God permeates every aspect of our lives. It affects our relationships. It affects what we think about ourselves. It affects our emotions. It affects our physical bodies.

Everything in our world that is not what we know as "God" by name is a reflection of God. Our emotions are a reflection of God. Our physicality is a reflection of God. Everything is intertwined, like the elements of Earth: land, sky, water. At some point each merges with and affects the other.

Ultimately, all forms of emotional and physical pleasure are but a shadow of our experience of God. Ultimately, all human desire lead to God. God is at the source of all human yearning. When we silence the droning demands of the ego, we can hear what our souls are really calling for.

God is the sweet nectar of ecstasy. When I experience a blissful orgasm as painful, at some level—and even if I'm not conscious of the fact—I'm experiencing my relationship with God as painful. Misperception is the source of pain.

Expanding the relationship with God can deepen and brighten the colors of our world, imbuing us with more joy and happiness than we thought could exist in our humble and hurting human hearts. We are God—collectively and individually. Ultimately, the relationship with God is the same as the relationship with ourselves—and everything around us.

Knowing God cannot be accomplished through just our minds, or just our emotions, or just our physical bodies. Our relationship with God requires the willingness of every part of us. God cannot be held within the limits of any comfort zone.

We all want a deeper experience of God—not theory, not hype, not mystification. And no one can do it for us, neither minister, nor saint, nor guru. Expanding our experiences of God can be discovered only from within.

Tantra does not give answers about God. Tantra only teaches us the skills we need that will allow us to find the answers within.

Tantra teaches us how to pull God into ourselves. When God is in our bodies and minds, we hear God, we know God, we embody God, to whatever degree our comfort zones can handle.

Tantra's ultimate gift can be a never-ending heightening of our experience of God. Our exploration of God can expand, deepen, and widen within our spiritual selves, just as the bodily pleasure of tantra slowly encompasses more and more of our physical selves.

The purpose within each session of tantra is to experience God. During the early years of tantra, my experience of God was limited and would last a few seconds now and then. Through consistent ritual, I grew to experience more and more moments of love, oneness, and God. The moments then became more profound. I have experienced God in ways I never knew possible—as though exercising the ultimate sense deep inside my soul, my God-sense, the sense that shines with a brightness more stunning than the sun.

God is always with us, it cannot be any other way. The only difference is whether or not we perceive it. What does it feel like when God is inside our bodies? When we viscerally feel his presence? There is a direct connection between kundalini's presence in the body and our consciousness of God. Sometimes it feels like the female aspect of God, the one that nurtures and gives us sustenance. When its warmth fires our creative impulses, we feel kundalini as the male aspect of God. When kundalini is awakened properly and in a balanced way, we cannot be conscious of anything but the relationship with God.

But why do I also experience pain? Why is kundalini not always comfortable? Why do I have an orgasm that seems to hurt? What is the underlying resistance that I keep stumbling over while walking down this spiritual path that is bringing me closer and closer to God?

Though I had increased my experience of God, I had not addressed some ugly doubts from my past. Now that the crack was exposed, I had to face this ultimate test.

My experience of God through tantra—in which I could feel God's essence in my heart and my partner's heart and deep within the cells of our bodies—was not the God of my past.

God of My Past

God was a subject of confusion during my childhood. God could mean many things, and if nothing else he was a puzzle to my curious mind. In fact, the fantastic intrigue and mystery are what fueled my search—at least in the beginning.

But what happens when God's novelty wears off? When the burning fire fades to glowing coal? When a few too many heartbreaks and disappointments get in the way of youthful idealism?

What did God mean to me?

By rote, I regurgitated the spiritually correct answers. God is love. God is all that is good. God is everything.

But let me be honest. In the deep dark corners of my mind lurked thoughts of which I am not particularly proud. This hidden part of me has an altogether different opinion about the almighty God.

God is sacrifice. God is hypocrisy. God is dominance over my free will. God is the ultimate oppressive authority figure, cast on us by oppressive society, out to squash my freedom and youth. God is death; I will not be united with him until I am buried. God can send me to hell. God is the puppeteer of the world, creating suffering and misery for punishment or amusement. God is a white-bearded male. Maybe there is no God.

My parents could never agree about God. Perhaps God caused their separation.

God was *my* bitter lemon.

The Chasm

I struggled with a semantic dichotomy that divides the religions of the East and West. It divided my past and present. It separated my tantric self from my Christian self. This issue revolved around the difference between illumination and enlightenment.

Illumination means "gnosis," or the "knowledge" of spiritual truth. Illumination is intellectual understanding.

Western religion generally embraces the concept of illumination. Christianity teaches that Jesus was *the* son of God—it's not as though there are multiple sons or daughters of God. One "superhuman" guy, who is part of the one and only Holy Trinity, saved us all, and the rest of us should be grateful, but it's not like we'll ever become as high up on the spiritual chain as Jesus. Jesus is not really our brother in the sense of equality. What are my options, then, as a Christian? I can gain illumination—knowledge—of the godly ways of Jesus and other saints by studying, and become more God-like through the performance of good deeds.

If I do that, true oneness with God will occur only after I have died. I can know God, and even act in God's likeness. But I cannot become one with God inside the boundaries of my skin. It is as though we cannot be one with God because of our physical nature. That leads me to believe that there is something unspiritual about our physical bodies.

As a Christian, I could know God mentally, but not physically.

Enlightenment, on the other hand, is the actual embodiment of oneness with God. Body and spirit are not mutually exclusive. Enlightenment happens inside the body, whether that moment occurs while mowing the lawn or on the deathbed.

Through the eyes of this philosophy, all saints, such as Buddha and Jesus, were ordinary people like you and me who achieved enlightenment. The whole idea of heaven and hell is turned inward—heaven and hell are inside us now, not a destination we will reach upon death. We do not need to die to be one with God.

Tantra was a major shift in my perception. I had no preconceived "bad" ideas of what the embodiment of God would "feel" like. In my Eastern-way infancy, I soaked up everything, unbiased.

But ultimately it led me back to me. Ultimately I had to face the mental part of me that knew God intellectually, in ways that seemed to scar my soul.

Deepening of the Chasm

In the eighth year of my tantric study, as my Western understanding of God collided with my tantric experience of God, the discomfort was almost unbearable. When I began to look more deeply at the problem, the pain increased, like a wound reacting from the medicine that could cause healing.

I was feeling resistance that went beyond my emotions. More, it felt as if it had to do with how my soul was feeling. The feeling was *spiritual pain*.

Spiritual pain feels much worse than a painful orgasm. Spiritual pain is when your soul hurts. It can be compared to emotional pain, such as sadness or grief, but it is not so acute. At the same time, it feels much deeper, as though penetrating beyond the present range of emotions that so often distracts us. Spiritual pain imparts the sense that we are acting against the grain of nature: against both our own grain and that of the universe.

It can occur from outside events that do not seem to follow the proper sequence of life, such as the unexpected death of a child. But it often occurs from our choices. When we act against our highest good, we increase spiritual pain. When we take a path or direction in life contrary to our purpose in life, spiritual pain is the result. It is the sense of dread that a woman who is not in love feels the night before her wedding.

Sometimes spiritual pain can take the form of illness or insomnia. Its voice can be conscience or intuition. In my case it was also kundalini, whose physical presence in my body brought to light everything I was trying to deny. I had immense pain in my stomach, for not acting on my inner principles, in my heart, for shutting out love, in my throat, for not speaking my truth, and in my head, for not listening to wisdom.

My spiritual pain had to do with my perception of God. And herein lay the biggest test of my life.

I wanted to leave my tantric path.

Oneness
with God

hat is really so heartbreaking is that God has been with me all along, and I simply avoided his presence. Yet now I can feel him inside my heart, as closely as I feel my partner. We are one now: his body speaks to mine, and I can hear. I can see what his mind visualizes; I can see the shiny, white light, with a tinge of yellow, like sunlight bursting a window, surrounding both of us. Our hearts are one, our hearts are made of the breath of God.

I wanted out. I itched to move on. I had many great reasons.

Maybe I've become codependent, I thought, as my family had warned me. Maybe this relationship with my partner is unhealthy. Isn't it high time that I give up my eccentric ways and abandon this tantric sexual relationship and settle down into a traditional, monogamous relationship? After all, I can't even talk about my spiritual path to most people I interact with. It certainly makes finding a boyfriend quite difficult. I don't want to be so different!

What about my desire to be a mother? What about a family? How can I possibly raise children when I follow this spiritual path? How would they fare with a mother so different from other mothers? And to find a man who wants tantra as much as I, and is in a position to be my lifelong partner, seems unlikely.

What about honoring my Christian upbringing? Who am I to forge a new way of experiencing God? Who am I to think I know more than the rest of my family?

These were the thoughts that dominated my consciousness. I didn't want to look any deeper. You see, I had become very strong as a result of progressing on this spiritual path. My logical mind was smart. I had become so strong, in fact, that logical justifications were easy to find. But they didn't drown out the soft voice inside me: the voice of the higher self that can't be reasoned away.

To avoid this voice, I tried desperately to find something that would pull me away: from the country, from life as I knew it, from everything. I just wanted out.

I worked very hard not to think about my spiritual pain. I kept a busy schedule. I worked long hours and socialized as much as possible. I avoided spending time alone. I stopped practicing tantra altogether. I cut down on doing my spiritual disciplines. I desperately flung myself into a relationship with a man who had no interest whatsoever in spirituality.

Agonizing months crept by. I tried to convince myself that I was doing the right thing. But everything got worse.

I began to lose my sense of identity and self-confidence. I became exceedingly shy and self-conscious, doubting every aspect of myself and my life. I reverted back to the low self-esteem I had as a young girl. My work suffered. I felt like a child during meetings with customers and was unable to communicate even the simplest of concepts. I began to find it hard to socialize because I was afraid that people would discover how insecure I was.

My spiritual pain manifested in several physical ways. I broke out in rashes that would not go away. I developed gastroesophogeal reflux disease and terrible insomnia.

I pretended to the world that I was choosing a new way in life. I was lying to myself.

To anyone who didn't know the lesson I was learning, leaving my path and getting on with a "normal" life would seem like a natural progression, even something good for me.

But those who really knew me saw me preparing to abandon my life-long purpose, my calling. In every crevice of my heart and soul, I knew this to be true. Abandoning my path would feel like throwing my own child off a cliff. And then jumping after.

I felt torn, wanting two opposing lives.

Facing the Truth

There would be no way to resolve this crisis without an extremely strong intention. I really had to get to the bottom of the crisis—not for God, nor for my tantric partner, but for me. Just for me.

By my own choice, then, with all the strength I had, I decided to take a small spiritual sabbatical. I took two weeks off from work, and canceled all social plans. I took all the disciplines I had learned over the past eight years and merged them into ten days of intensive cleansing. I fasted on lemon water, tea, and a small amount of fruit juice. I meditated several times a day and also practiced kriya yoga. I wrote all of my thoughts, both good and bad, in a journal. I went on short walks to feel the sun on my face. I sat in front of the fire and looked deeply into its flames, asking for guidance and understanding.

It was during these ten days that I discovered the real reasons that I wanted to leave the tantric path. One was simply the pattern of time. I was in the womb for exactly eight months. The number eight stimulated my pattern to leave. But there were other agendas that my unconscious mind was trying hard to keep suppressed.

I doubted my very ability to be strong enough to stay on this path. I doubted my ability to commit. I didn't really think I could do it. I chose my spiritual path at the age of nineteen. Although a legal adult, in my heart I still felt like a child. I didn't take full responsibility for my decisions. Despite all my success, part of me still wanted to be a little girl. I still wanted to be taken care of. Maybe I felt that I had never been taken care of properly as a child, and somehow the world still owed that to me. Tantra, of course, is all about self-responsibility. I was afraid of responsibility. Doing what some-one told me to do was much easier than making my own choices. I didn't think I could do it all on my own.

I realized that when I first began this spiritual path, I thought I had wanted enlightenment and to feel nothing but love every moment of the day. Then I began to review all the pleasures that my spiritual path had brought up to now. Materially I had created great prosperity, security, independence, and the respect of my family and friends. Emotionally, I had gained high self-esteem and self-confidence and enjoyed positive and supportive relationships. Physically, I felt incredibly vibrant, sexual and innocent at the same time, with the ability to achieve orgasm for hours on end. Spiritually, I felt much more connected to God, and this nectar of kundalini served as a constant reminder. But had I achieved enlightenment?

Of course not. Yet if enlightenment were my true intention, why would I want to leave the path now?

Because, you see, enlightenment was not my real agenda. What I really wanted was all of the material, emotional, and physical things I had gained over the years. My ego was willing to let me change just enough for me to get all these great things in my life—but once I got them, what would be the need for God?

After spending so many years in faithful service to God, it was time to serve myself. I wanted things my way. I wanted to rebel. How much did I really want God to guide me?

This rebellion tied in to a deeper belief, which was that some part of me felt that who I am is separate from God. This thought was different from my occasional feeling that I'm separate from God—a normal feeling that occurs simply because I'm not spending my entire day in meditative contemplation. This thought was deeper, and the difference was that I knew this lie to be true. With total certainty, in the deep recesses of my soul, I believed that everything about me was separate from God.

I was afraid of knowing myself more. If I kept looking inside, perhaps I would discover that after all this time and effort, my essence was ugly, and black, and terrible.

On the flip side of this fear was that I *could be* one with God. I was afraid of losing my individuality. I was afraid of merging into nothingness, never to return to my soul as I know it—just merging into some awful indistinct blob.

I had really just started to open my heart during tantra. Fear of intimacy was still there to some degree. Somehow, in the past, I had been strong enough to overcome this fear to some extent to continue tantra. But now, every time I practiced tantra I felt increasingly more soft, open, and loving. I felt the whole context of my personality on the verge of shifting from self-centered to heart-centered. I was afraid that being so open and loving would hurt me. I was afraid of losing control. Still deeper was my fear that I would be hurt. When had I adopted the idea that if I open my heart, I get hurt?

I had mastered these deep pains just enough to get everything I wanted out of life. But where did I want to go now?

Becoming conscious of our own hidden agendas is one of the most powerful tools for transformation. It all comes back to the simple adage "Know thyself." When I finally admitted what all this resistance was about, both my emotional pain and my physical ailments began to diminish. Outwardly, I seemed pretty much the same to people. But inwardly I had grown up.

My spiritual path *is* me—it's not separate from me. And wherever I go, there I am. I am one with God. I am my path. My path is God. All are the same. I do have free will. I alone can even change my karmic destiny. I can leave my tantric path at any time. But what would be the point? I can never leave myself. Ultimately, the tantric path—my teachers, my tantric partner, my philosophies—mean nothing. Even if all of these things decided to leave me, I would still have my path within me.

There is a reason that tantra contains within it so many contradictions. Ultimately, it negates even itself. Everything in this world is temporal. The only thing we take with us is the relationship we have with God, with ourselves, and with other people—and these are ultimately the same thing. The path is love. And no matter how hard any of us tries, we can never leave our source, which is God. There is no other truth.

Spiritual paths of celibacy, in both Eastern and Western cultures, teach their members to want nothing, to be happy with what they have, and to devote their lives to the service of God. In other words, we are taught not to look at what we want but instead to see who we really are.

Now that I had everything I could possibly want in life, it would be easy to quit. It is always easier to be negative rather than positive, to destroy than to build up, to give up than to keep going. But what is a life lived without purpose of soul? What is a life lived full of regret for all the things we were too afraid to do?

The biggest test I faced was that now I must change my deepest motivations, from being self-centered to following a heart-centered path of service and devotion. I had chosen tantra partly because it would solve these material problems, these everyday issues I had in so many areas of my life. My motivation was primarily fear-based.

In Christianity we learn that being good will get us into heaven. We also see the same thing in different packaging in Eastern religions, in which being good will give us good karma and hence a better next life.

I had to ask myself a pivotal question: Do I want oneness with God simply for oneness with God, without any other benefits? Am I willing to give up all my attachments that are centered on fear and a sense of lack? Am I willing to love simply for the sake of love?

Transcending self-centered motivations means being good because it's the right thing to do, because it's our intrinsic nature, and because we see that it's who and what we are. This is oneness with self.

I began to meditate on really knowing that center of light within my heart. I could feel many contradictions and fears. I went beyond these fears, deeper. And that yearning—my yearning to be truly one with self and hence with God, to dissolve all desire into the singular desire for God—it was there all along! Since I was a very young child, it was there. Yes, I knew it would be scary to continue to venture into the unknown of self, the unknown of absolute truth, the unknown of constant bliss. I would need faith and courage.

Intentions

The core around which our spiritual self rotates, like electrons around a nucleus, has to do with intention. Intention determines the range of the spiritual comfort zone. Intention defines the ability to surrender and grow. Intention silhouettes the intimate relationship with God.

We should always know our intentions, for they are not as obvious as they appear. The more we know ourselves, the more we will know our true intentions. Not always do we have the best of intentions.

Often we look at life from the perspective of: "How can this benefit me?" This is a natural and normal reaction. But true happiness will find its way into our hearts when we ask instead, "What can I give?"

A spiritual path, despite all its wonderful benefits, is indeed a spiritual path. The purpose of tantra is spiritual, to improve the ultimate relationship—and that is with God.

Pursuing my spiritual path without the ultimate intention of growing my oneness with God resulted in partial happiness and partial success. It had its benefits, to be sure. It had brought rewards and gifts. But to limit my intentions to being fear-based caused me eventually to hit the wall. Whenever I pursued intentions that did not have at their core the ultimate desire for union with God, I would be unsatisfied on some level.

We each have within us an innate desire to become one with God. And desire is ultimately the reflection of the desire for God. When we are not aware of this, and focus our energies in limiting directions, then the fulfillment of desire becomes stale and hollow.

We will find everlasting happiness when we let go of all intentions that are not in alignment with developing our relationship with God. If we can't agree to such a commitment, we can begin to open the gates of joy by first wanting to make it our intention to improve and expand our relationship with God.

It was in this realization that I discovered that my spiritual journey had only just begun.

Integration 18

eyond pleasure. We have delved into hidden realms of our brain's happy juices and they poured forth in abundance. I can see, with my vision, the chakra of his heart! Floating just in front of his chest, it is the shape of a flower. Are my eyes deceiving me, or do I really see his spiritual heart? We complete each other's thoughts. He looks so young in the candlelight as I climb onto him, breathing it into my heart and pushing it down through my yoni into him, up into his lotus-shaped heart. This flow, we both feel it. Tonight we bask in our love for each other.

Tantra is a mother. Gentle and nurturing, silently wise, she shines the light of truth upon the dark illusions burdening our minds. She is the caretaker of Earth, for thousands of years patiently guiding us to our truth. Tantra is a child. Demanding our attention, she brings us infinite joy when we offer our abundant love. She knows simply that God feels good. Tantra is a father. He protects our innocence, defends our self-respect, and insists on purity in our actions.

Tantra seeks to open the heart. Within our hearts reside the pinnacle of every human desire. Our hearts are our inseparable link to God. Knowing this, we will never want.

Many wondrous things have happened on my way to knowing my heart. Most important, my sense of spirituality expands daily. Tantra stimulates energies within my body that help me feel God's presence. My kundalini has awakened, its delicious juices elevating my spirit with each phase of the Moon. I have learned faith, patience, and trust. I have learned integrity, honesty, and being good for good's sake.

I have learned to know my hidden agendas, the dark needs of my ego that can lie dormant but poised to destroy my higher purpose. I learned not to fear my shadows that are built of separation and doubt. I learned that oneness with God is not a destination but rather a path walked in the moment of now.

Tantra can be combined with our existing spiritual beliefs and values. We should let it gently add to our lives, and not give up what's most important. There is no official textbook or instruction manual for tantra. There are excellent books about tantra on the market, but these are personal interpretations and should be viewed as guidelines only. If we give tantra a manual, we will turn it into a religion that teaches dogma and behavior. Tantra is not a religion, and it is not about doctrine or dogmas. A spiritual path must be an individual path.

We should also combine tantra with other spiritual disciplines. Because tantra will awaken energies within us, by and through our sexuality, we will need other practices to help maintain balance and focus. Meditation disciplines our minds so that our consciousness grows along with our physical awakening and will also allow us to strengthen our intentions.

The one sacrifice that tantra asks is that we change everything within us that is not in our best interest. We must let go of everything that resists love. Every negative thought about ourselves and every negative feeling we have about the world around us: these must be surrendered.

A tantric awakening means gaining mastery of the emotions. All negative emotion, when projected toward others, is like a spinning wheel. It does nothing to address the source of the issue, and it hurts only us. We must always look within. Turning the other cheek is easy when we see the God in ourselves, for then we will see the God in others. Turning the other cheek means affirming that it doesn't matter what others do because we see their divinity, beyond their actions.

A tantric awakening means taking responsibility for all emotions and choices. Conscious choice is the surest way to have no regret. Our society has adopted the bad habit of blame and victimization. We want someone or something to come and save us from ourselves. But being a victim inevitably makes us feel terrible, because we know, deep down, that we are more than this. We really want to create our own destinies. The time for nursing our wounds is over. It is time to take rightful ownership of our full power.

A tantric awakening means gaining the courage to know what we really want and then to act on that desire. We will discover internal agendas that do not serve our highest good. The key is to become conscious of these agendas and instead surrender to the soul's desire. We are much more than our negative emotions, our personal lies, the petty games we play. We are much more than our judging and self-condemning minds would have us believe. Heart strength means knowing, with quiet confidence, that we are pure divinity. We are talented, beautiful, and unique children of God.

My intimate relationship with tantra, now having surpassed the decade mark as I turn thirty this year, has just started to unfold. There is much for me to learn, for I am still learning to combine my heart with my sexuality. I am still understanding my relationship with myself, with others, and with God. I am still learning how to be a better friend, lover, and daughter. I have yet to discover what it means to be a mother and wife. But this tantric awakening, however ecstatic, has just begun.

Tantric Organizations and Contact Information

For more information on how to start your own tantric practice or to participate in a workshop, you may wish to contact one of the reputable organizations listed below.

Tantrika International, founded by Bodhi Avinasha. Bodhi is a leading teacher of tantra today, and creator of Ipsalu Tantra. She taught with Sunyata Saraswati, coauthored the leading tantric text, *Jewel in the Lotus,* was a student of Osho, and is in communication with Babaji.
12115 Magnolia Blvd., Valley Village, CA 91607, (818) 487-5725.

Source School of Tantra, established by Charles and Caroline Muir. The Muirs have been teaching for many years. PO Box 1451, Wailuku, Hawaii 96793, (808) 243-9851.

Skydancing Tantra Institute, founded by Margot Anand. PO Box 1192, Cobb, CA 95426, Toll-Free 1-877-982-6872.

Feedback for the author can be directed to valeriebrooks@socal.rr.com, or visit www.tantranow.com.

BOOKS OF RELATED INTREST

Desire
The Tantric Path to Awakening
by Daniel Odier

The Complete Kama Sutra
The First Unabridged Modern Translation of the Classic Indian Text
Translated by Alain Daniélou

The Illustrated Kama Sutra • Ananga-Ranga • Perfumed Garden
Translated by Sir Richard Burton and F. F. Arbuthnot

Sexual Secrets: Twentieth Annivesary Edition
The Alchemy of Ecstasy
by Nik Douglas and Penny Slinger

Tantric Quest
An Encounter with Absolute Love
by Daniel Odier

Celtic Sex Magic
For Couples, Groups, and Solitary Practitioners
by Jon G. Hughes

The Sexual Teachings of the White Tigress
Secrets of the Female Taoist Masters
by Hsi Lai

Sacred Sexuality in Ancient Egypt
The Erotic Secrets of the Forbidden Papyrus
by Ruth Schumann Antelme and Stéphane Rossini

Inner Traditions • Bear & Company
P.O. Box 388
Rochester, VT 05767
1-800-246-8648
www.InnerTraditions.com

Or contact your local bookseller